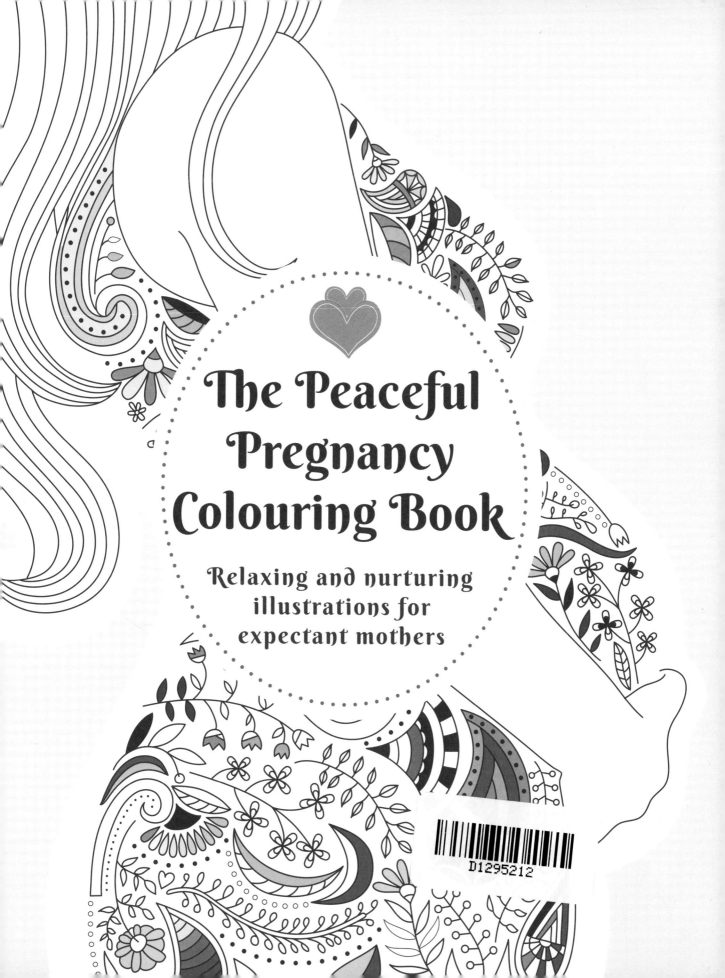

The Peaceful Pregnancy Colouring Book

Relaxing and nurturing
illustrations for
expectant mothers

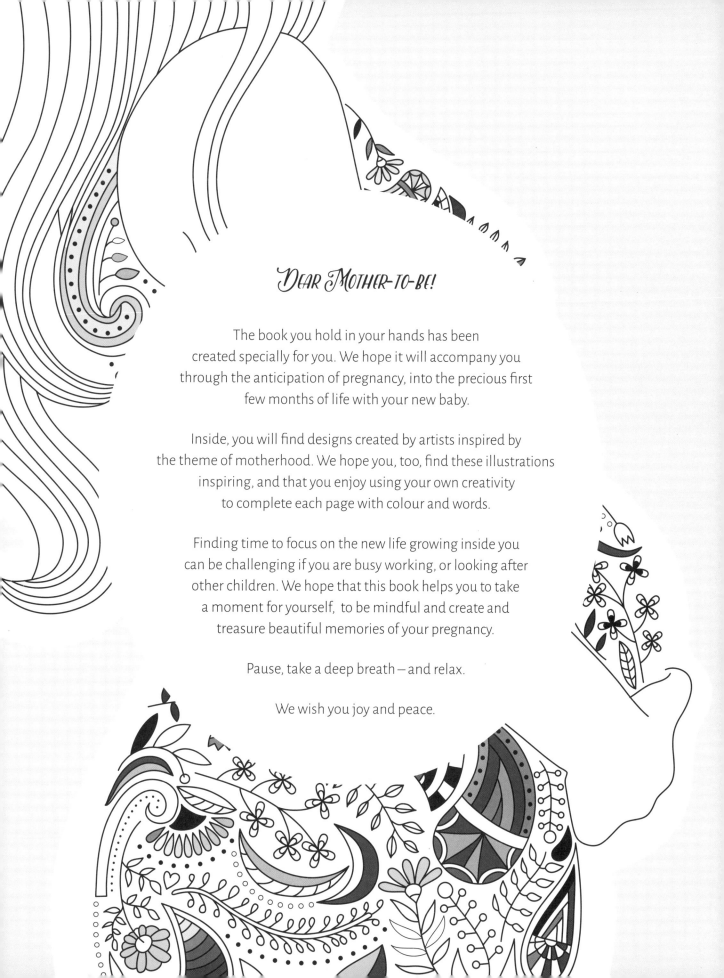

Dear Mother-to-be!

The book you hold in your hands has been
created specially for you. We hope it will accompany you
through the anticipation of pregnancy, into the precious first
few months of life with your new baby.

Inside, you will find designs created by artists inspired by
the theme of motherhood. We hope you, too, find these illustrations
inspiring, and that you enjoy using your own creativity
to complete each page with colour and words.

Finding time to focus on the new life growing inside you
can be challenging if you are busy working, or looking after
other children. We hope that this book helps you to take
a moment for yourself, to be mindful and create and
treasure beautiful memories of your pregnancy.

Pause, take a deep breath — and relax.

We wish you joy and peace.

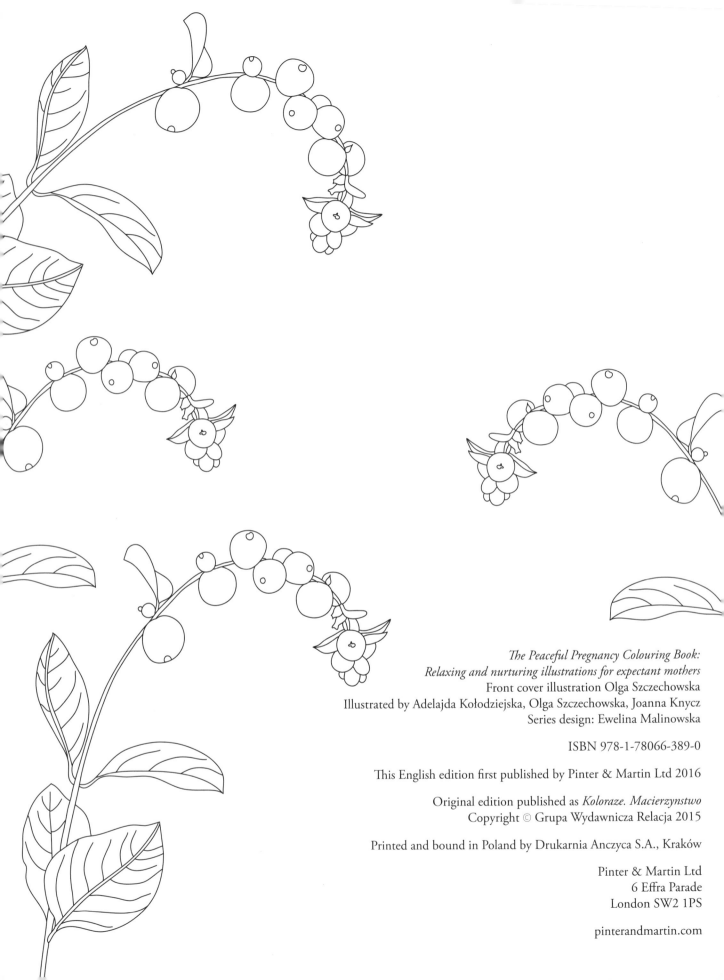

The Peaceful Pregnancy Colouring Book:
Relaxing and nurturing illustrations for expectant mothers
Front cover illustration Olga Szczechowska
Illustrated by Adelajda Kołodziejska, Olga Szczechowska, Joanna Knycz
Series design: Ewelina Malinowska

ISBN 978-1-78066-389-0

This English edition first published by Pinter & Martin Ltd 2016

Original edition published as *Koloraze. Macierzynstwo*
Copyright © Grupa Wydawnicza Relacja 2015

Printed and bound in Poland by Drukarnia Anczyca S.A., Kraków

Pinter & Martin Ltd
6 Effra Parade
London SW2 1PS

pinterandmartin.com

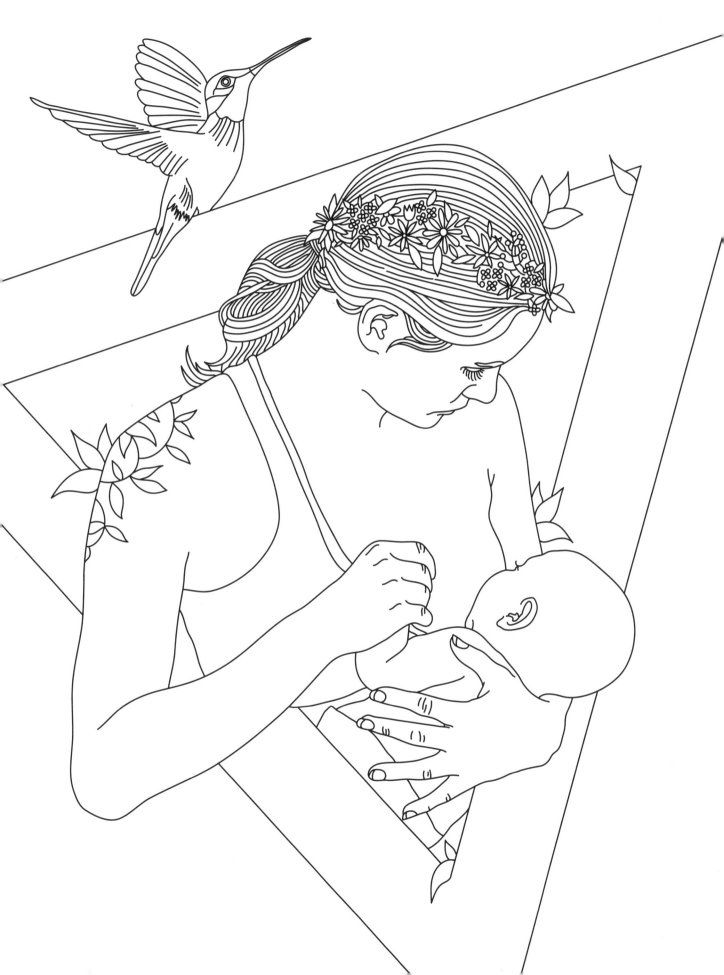

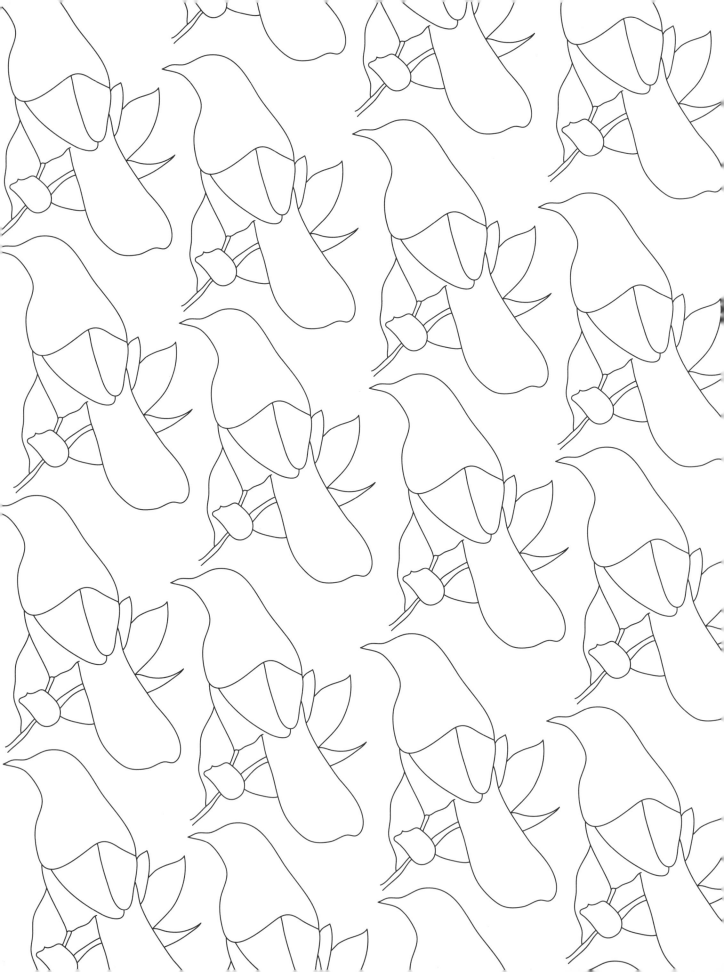

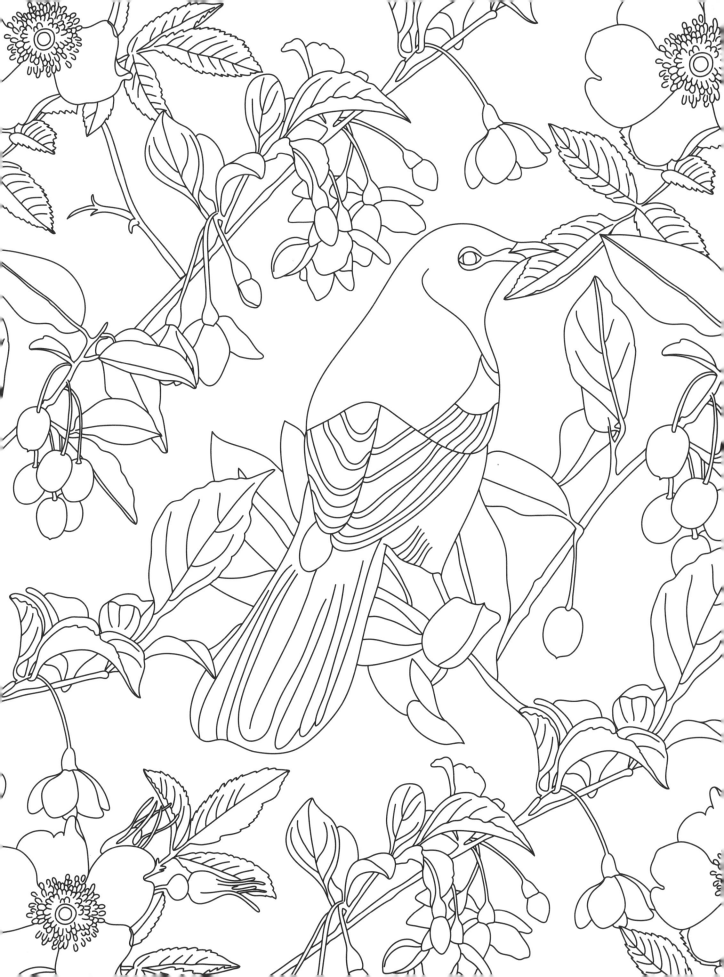

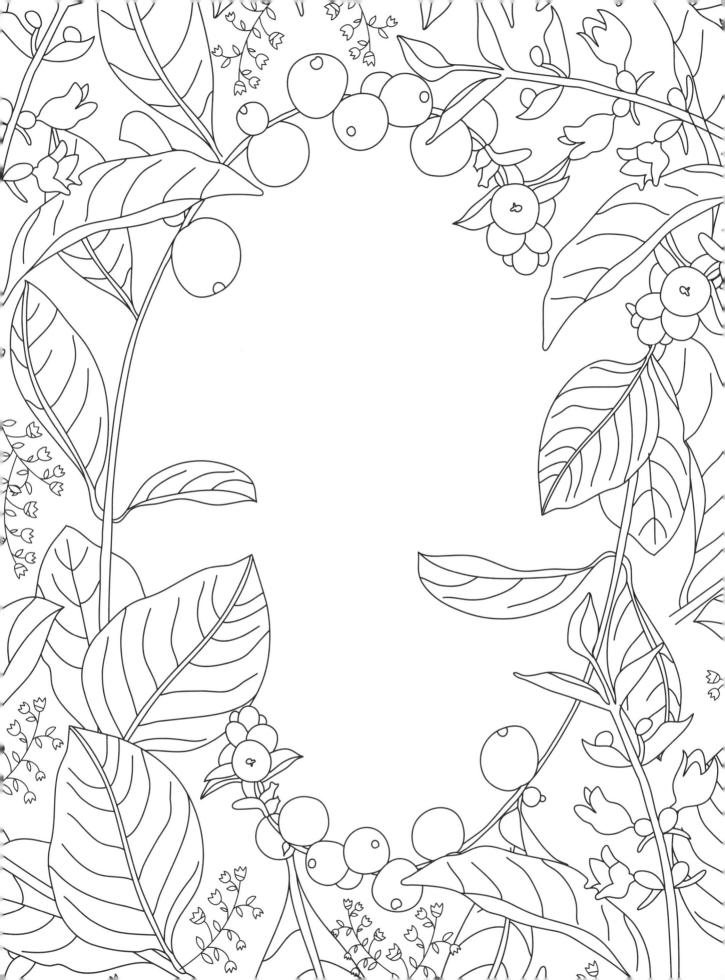

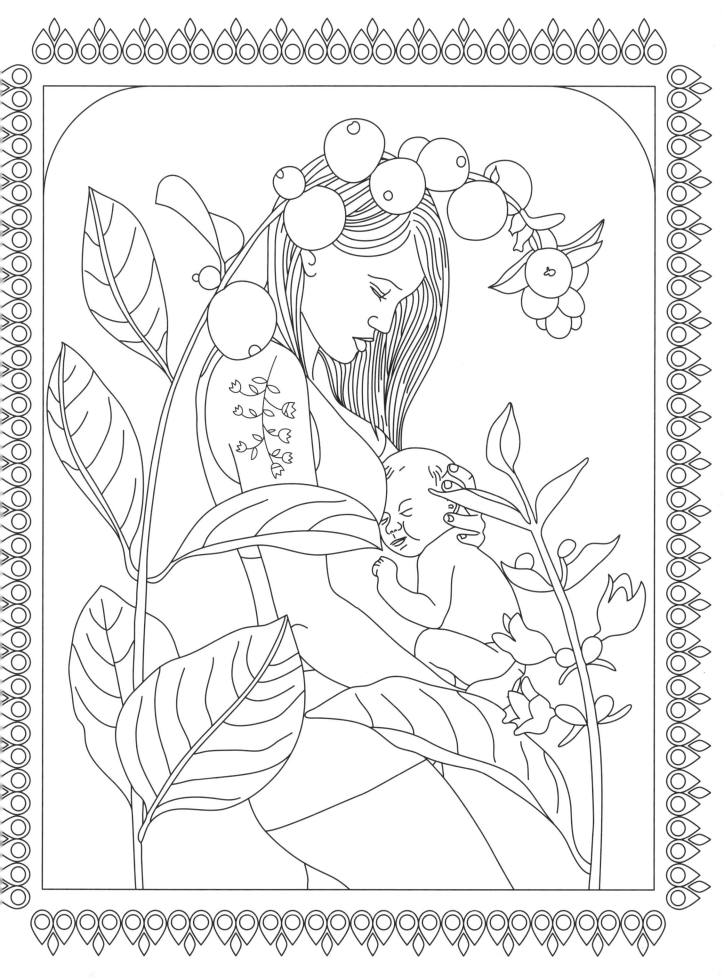

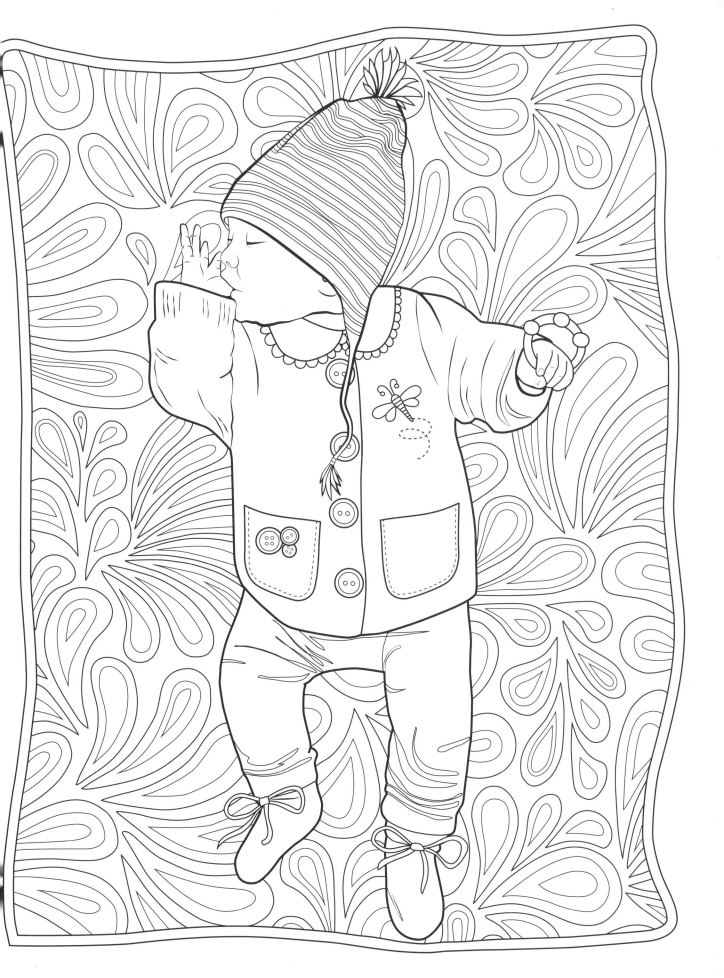

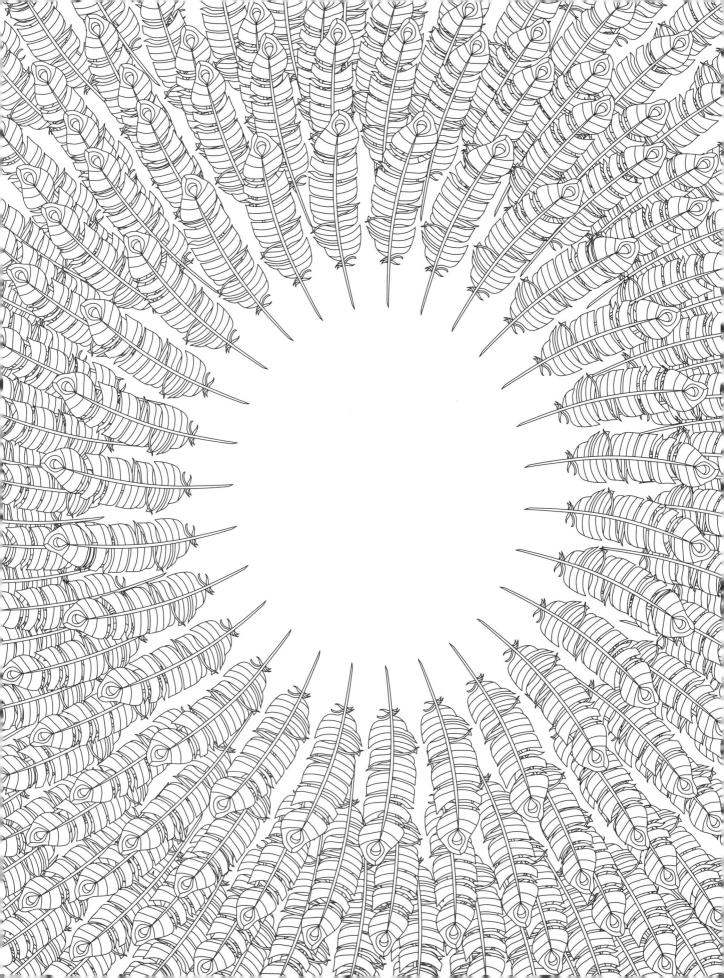

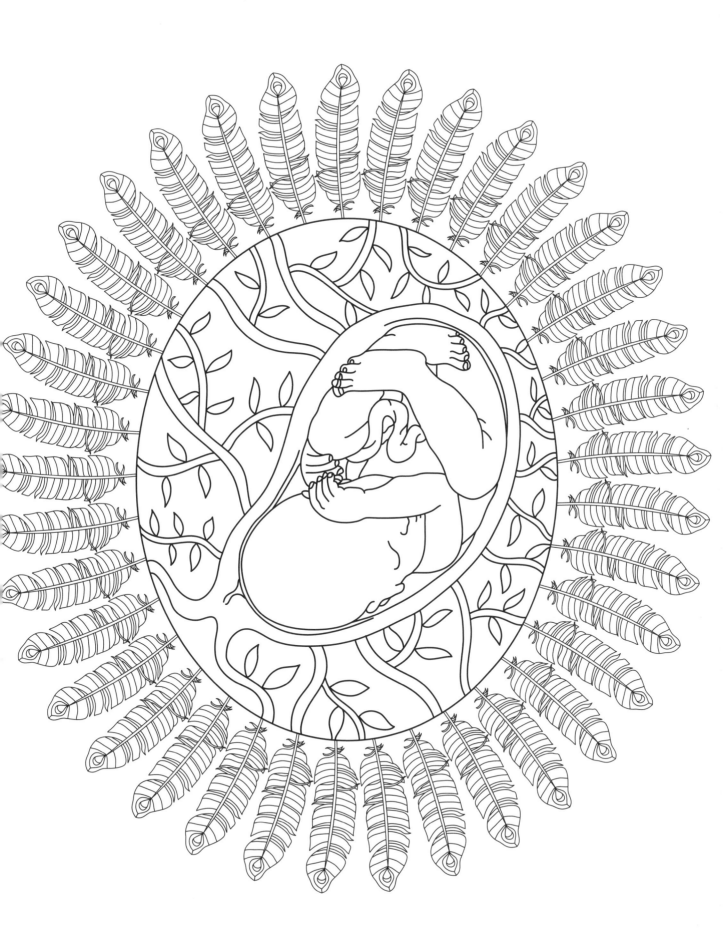

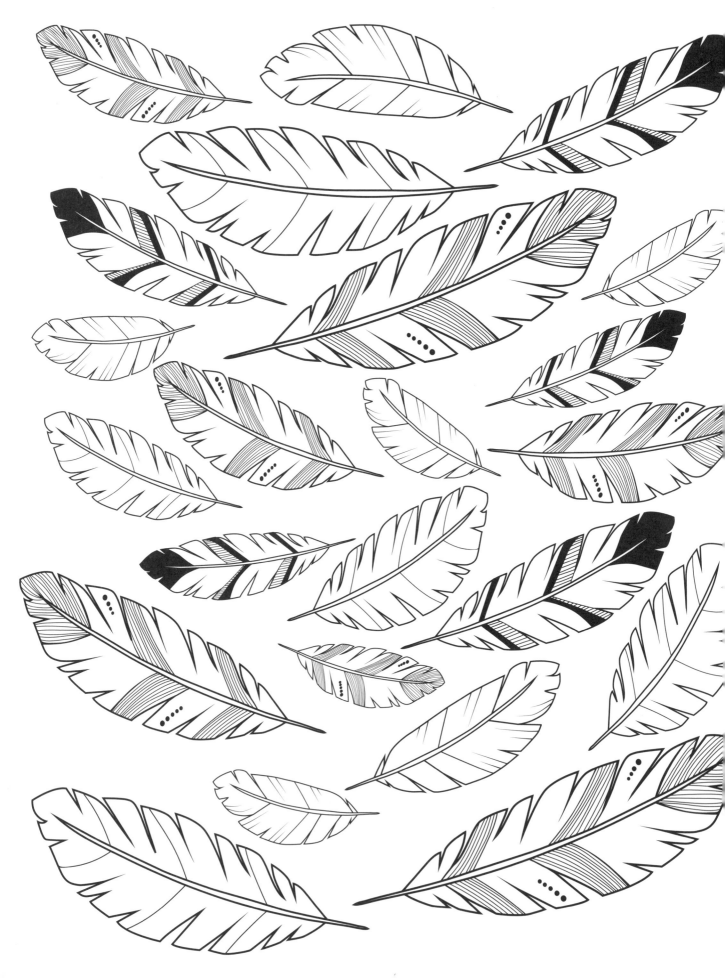

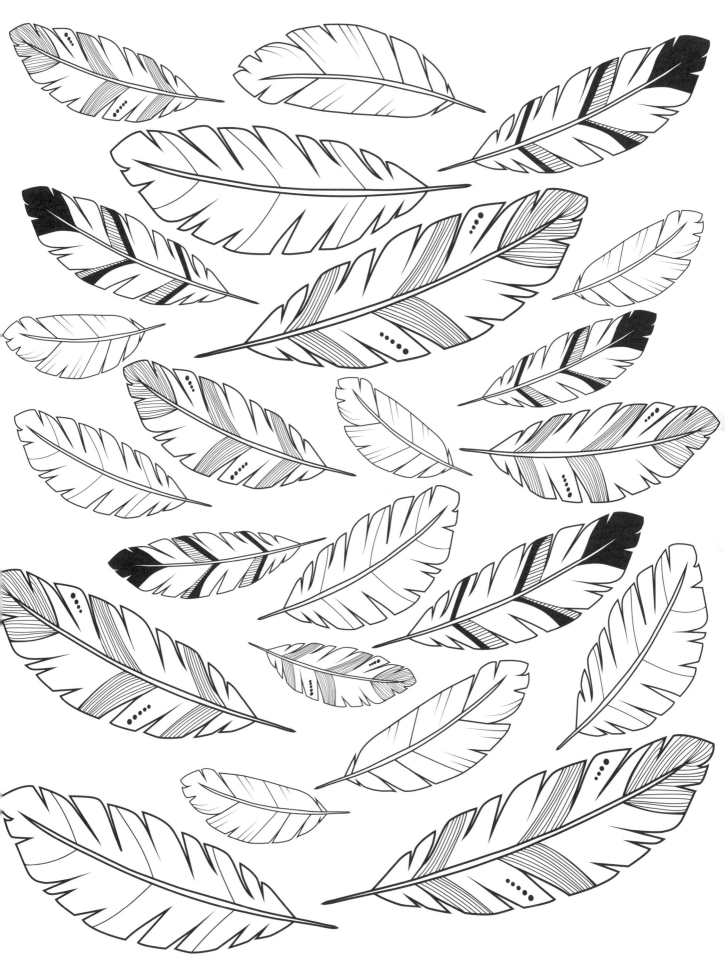

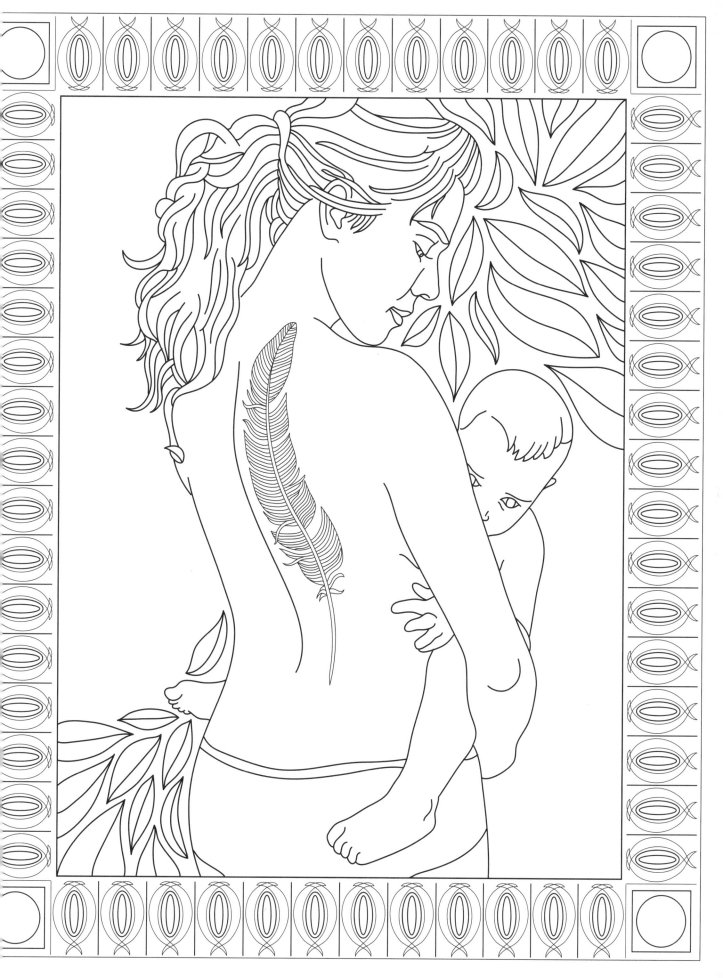

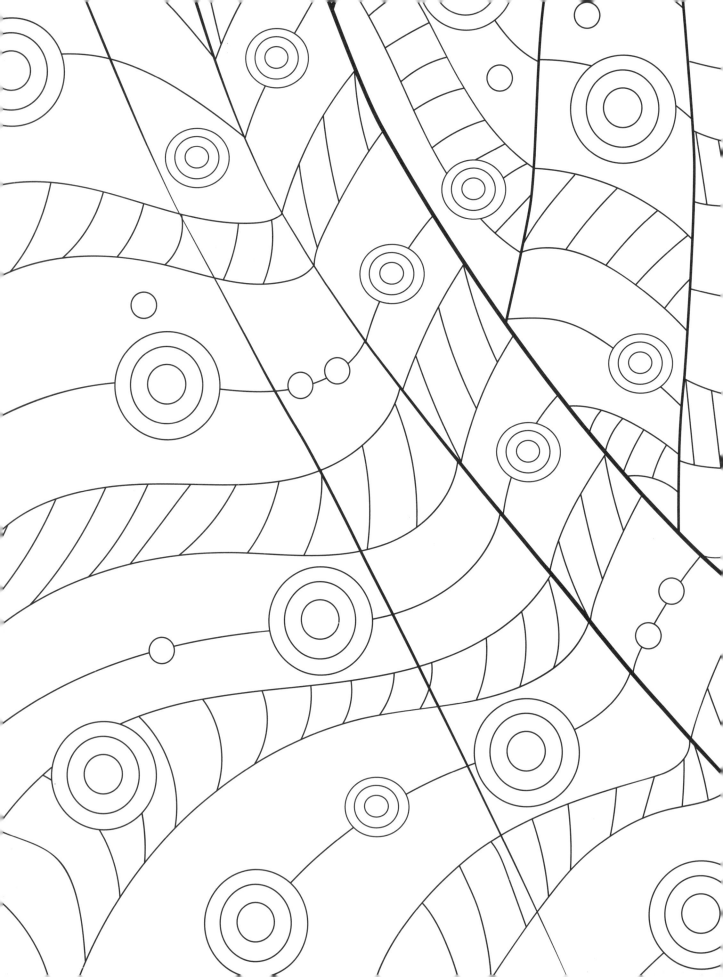

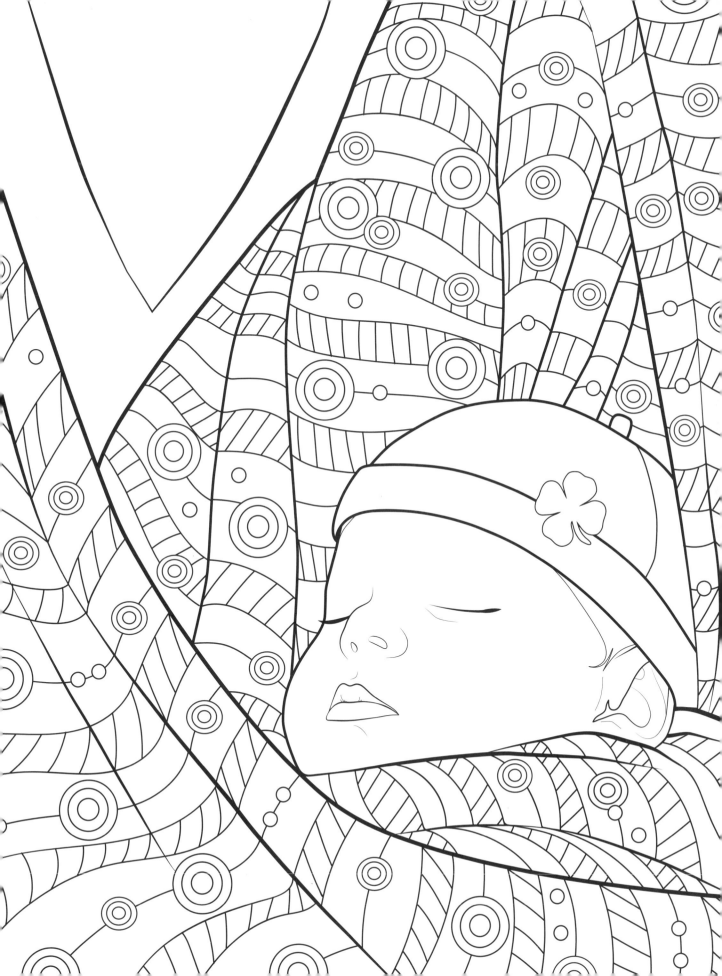

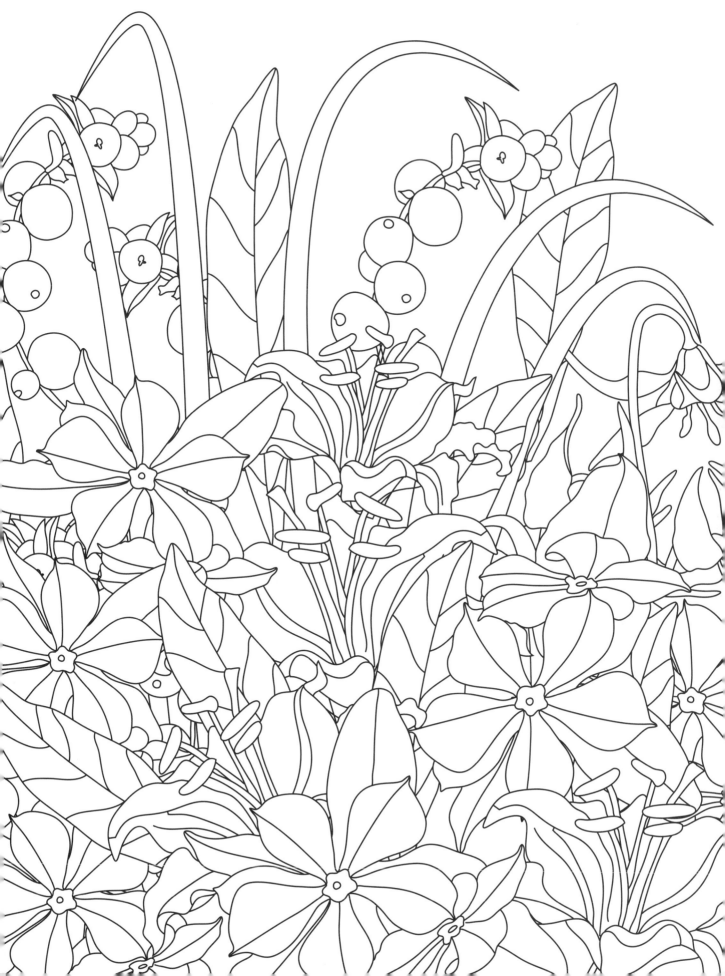

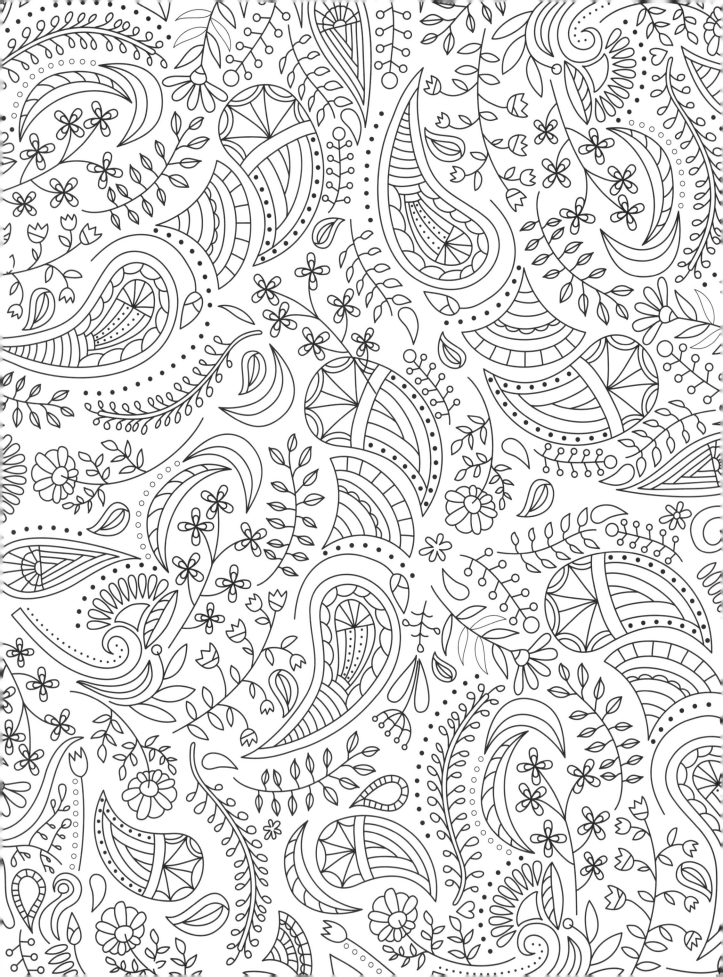

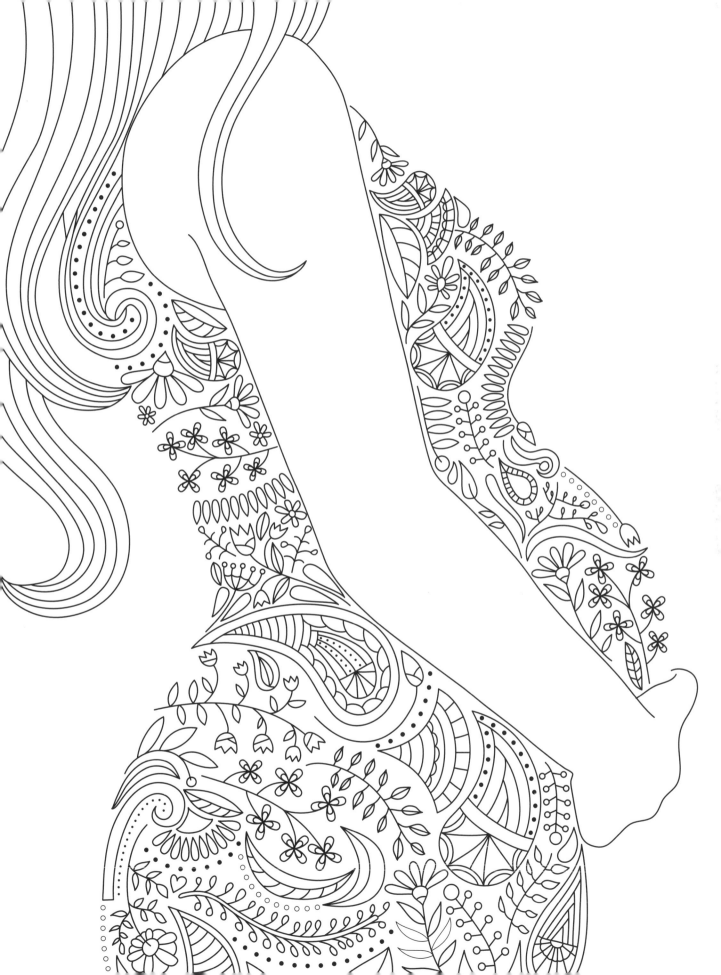

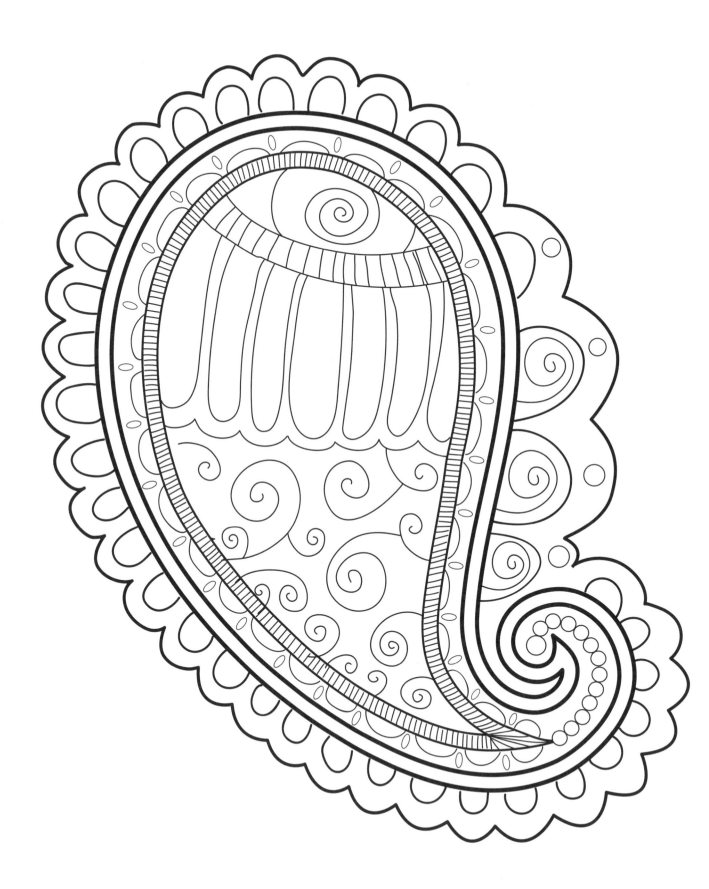

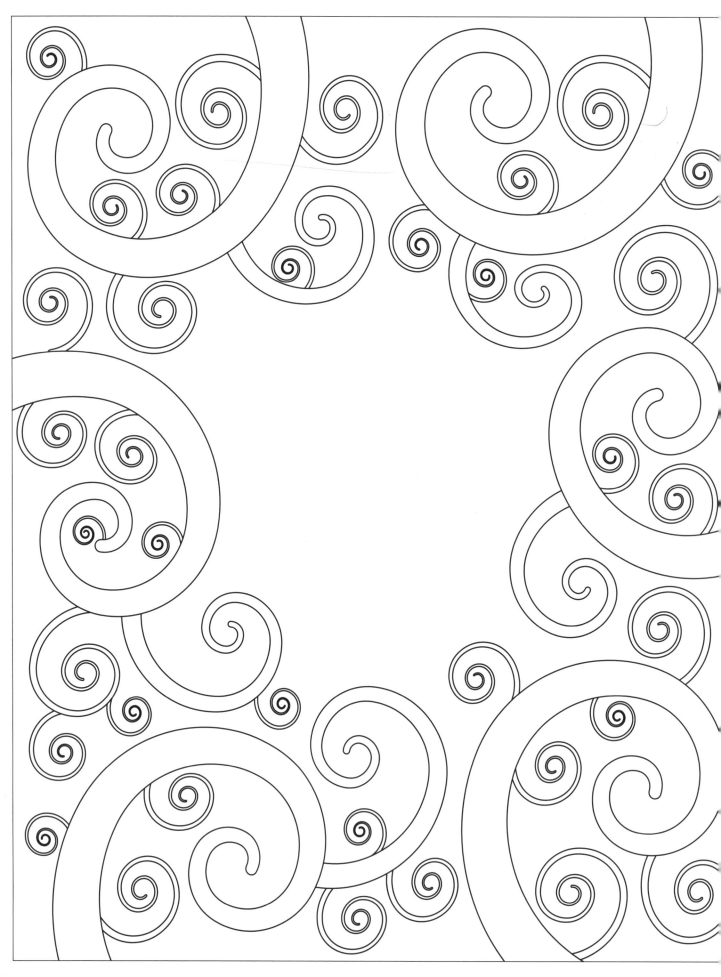

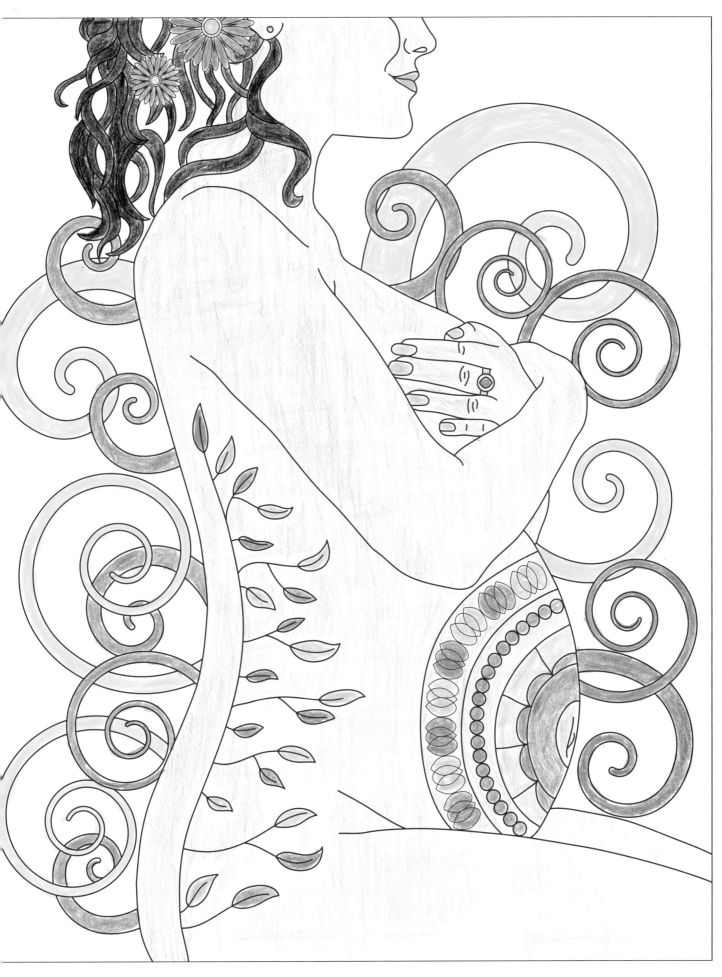

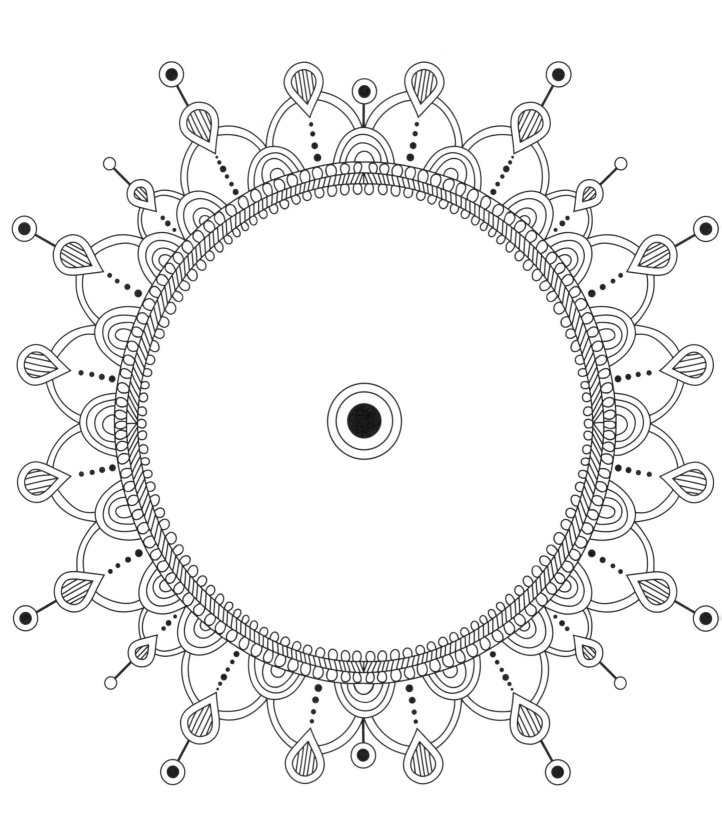

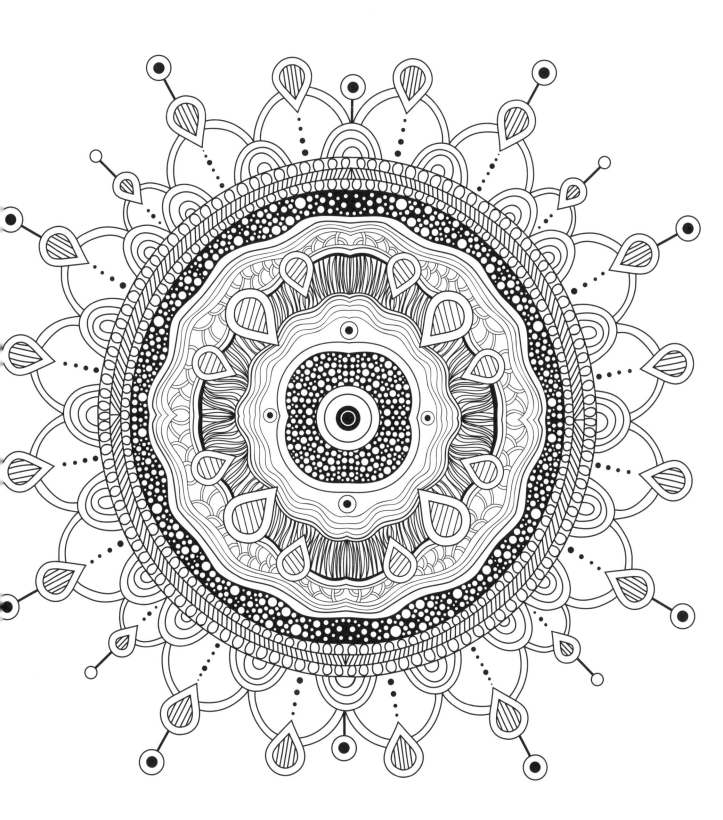

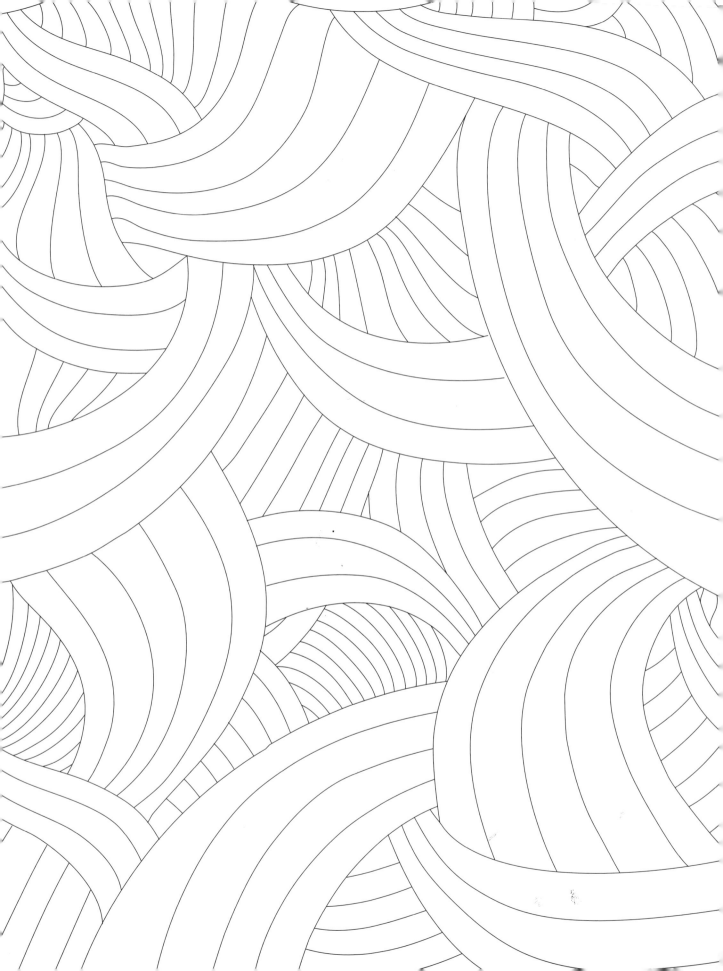

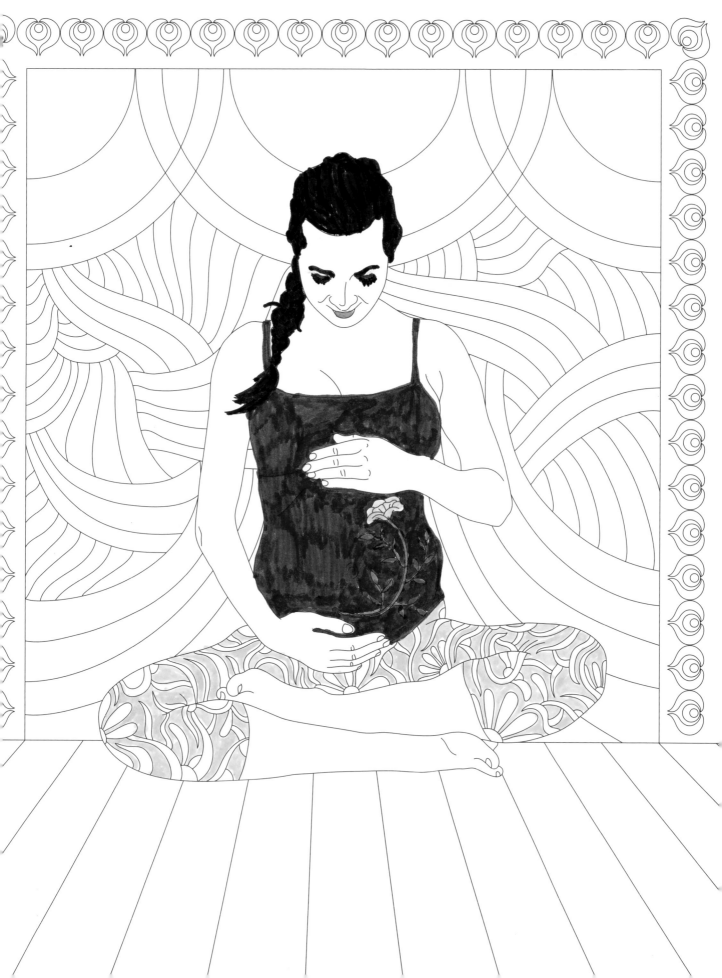

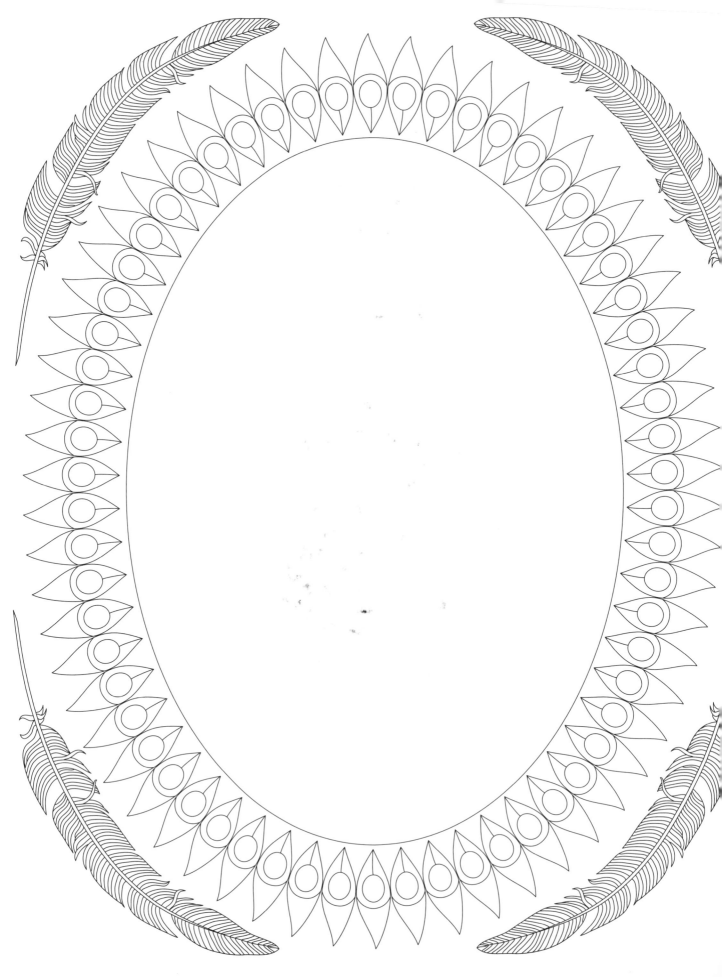

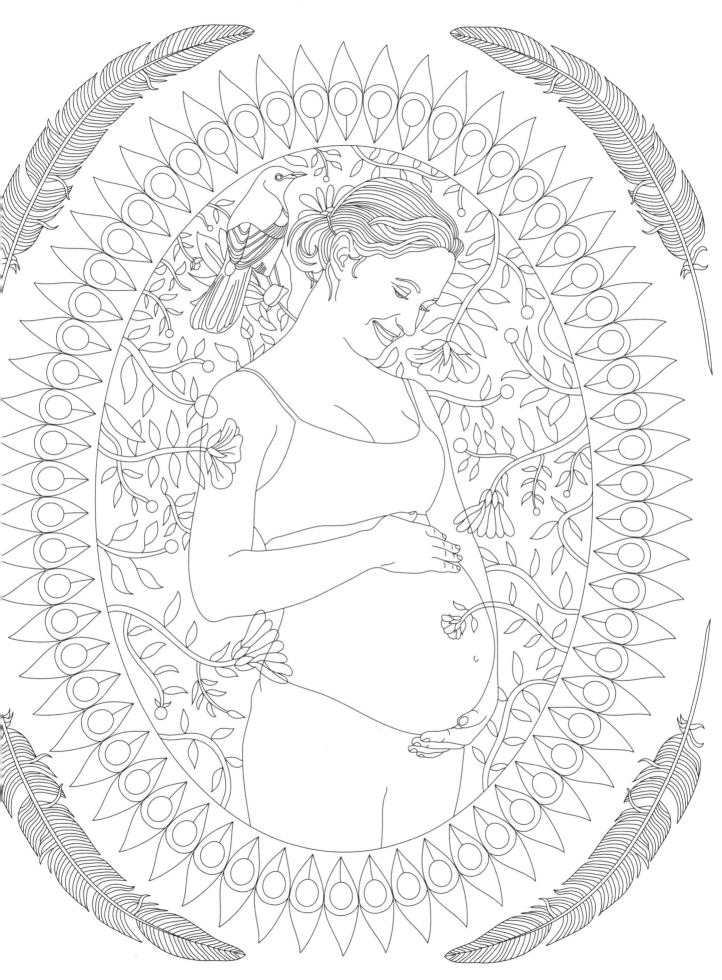

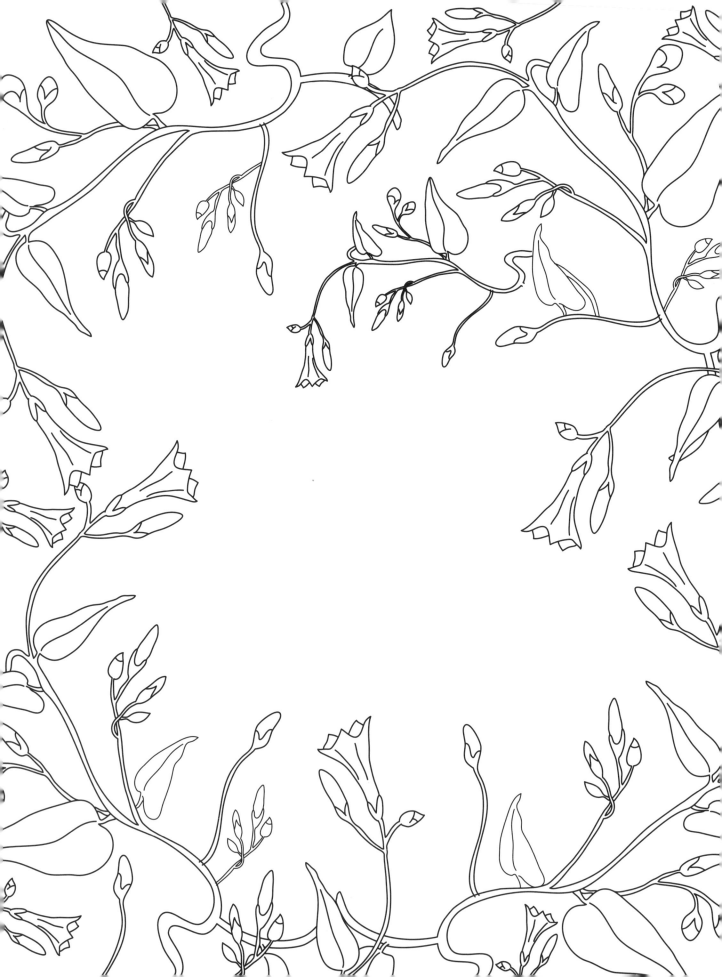

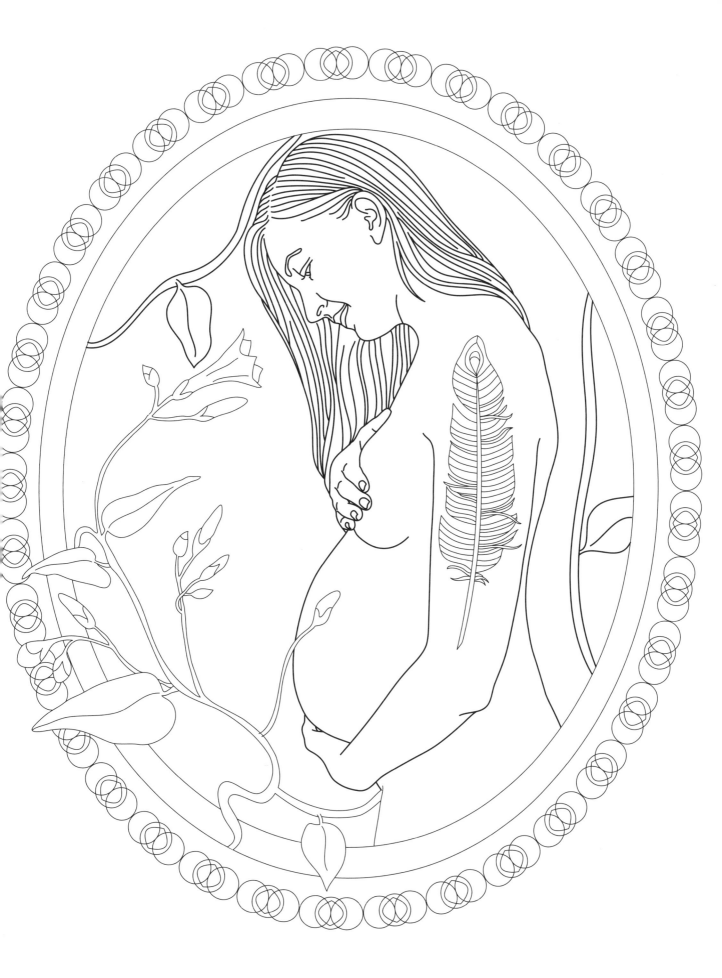

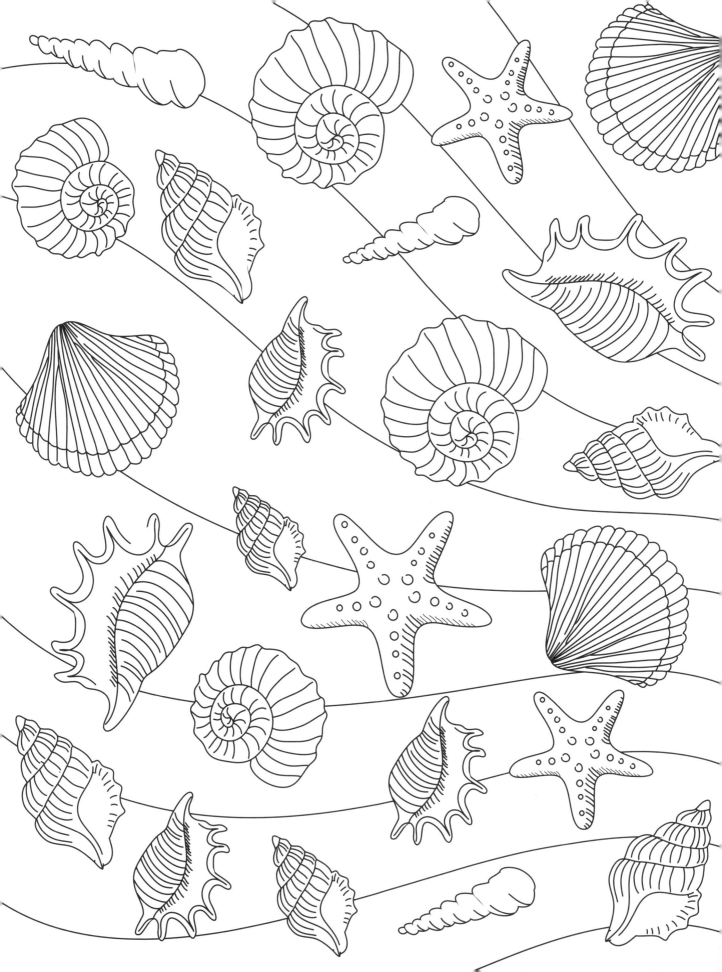

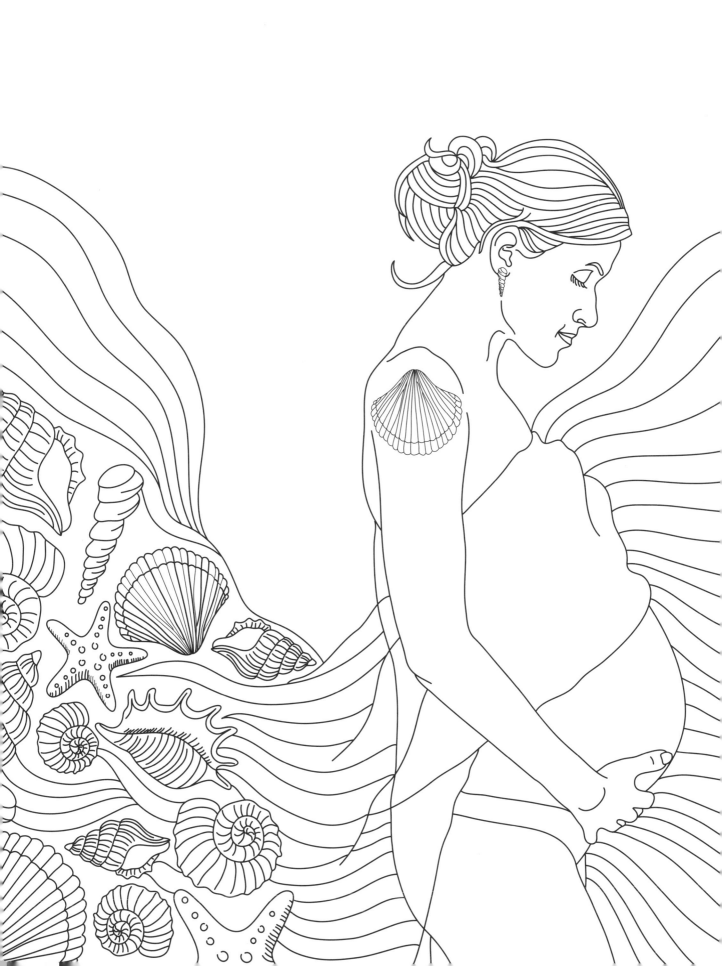

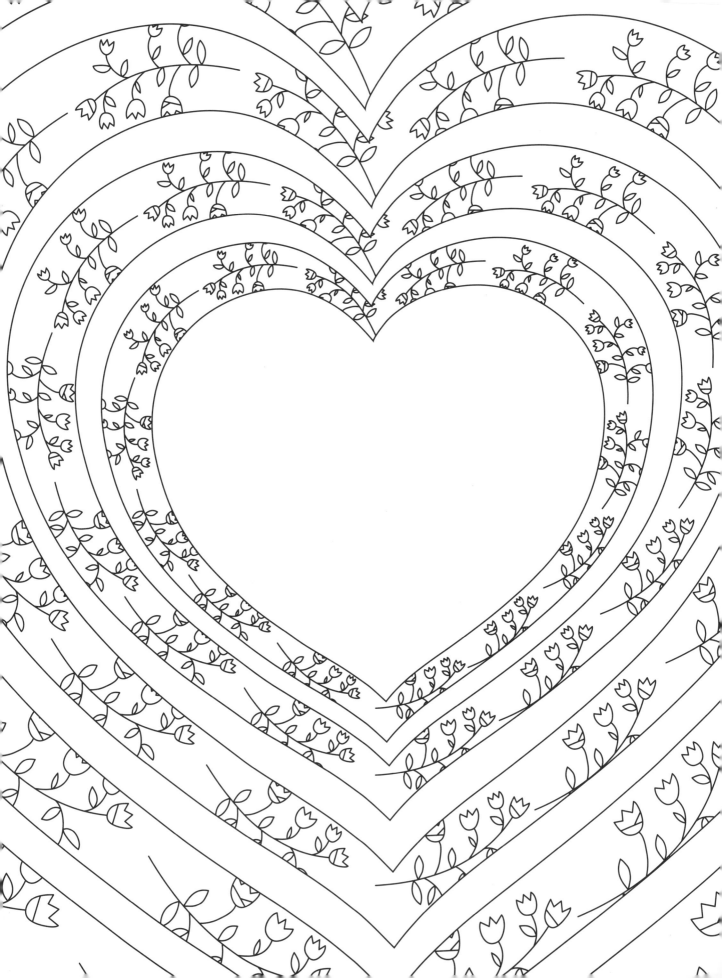

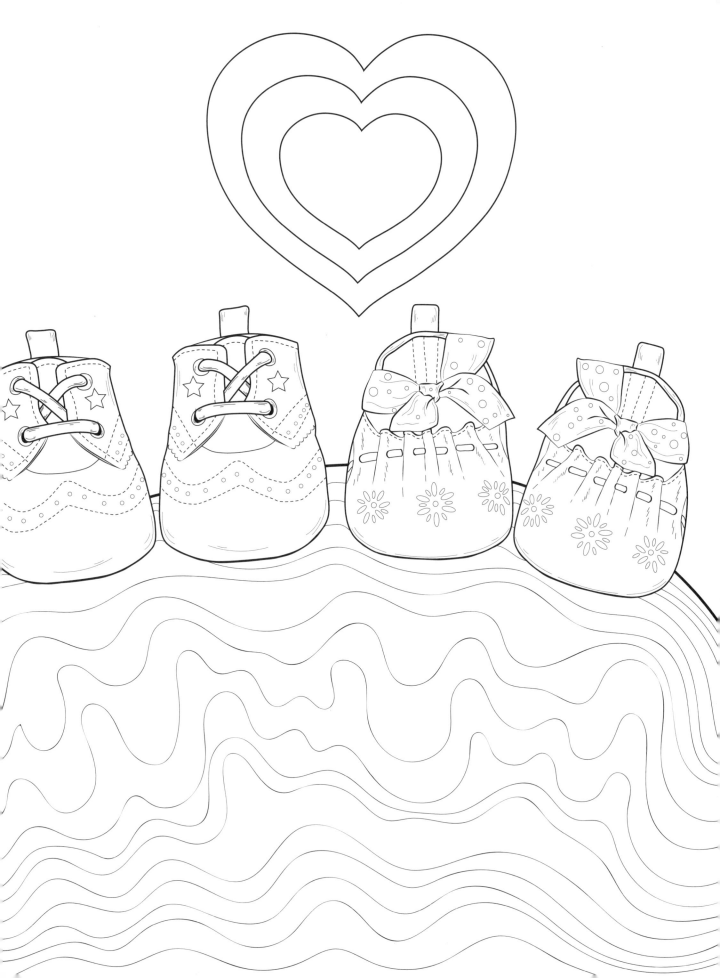

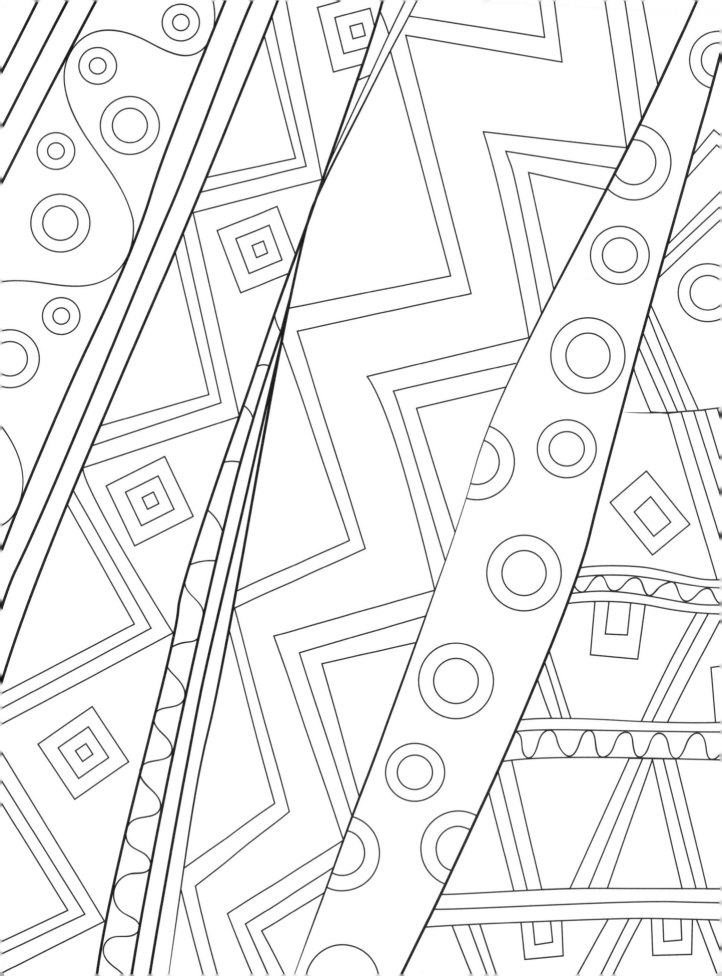

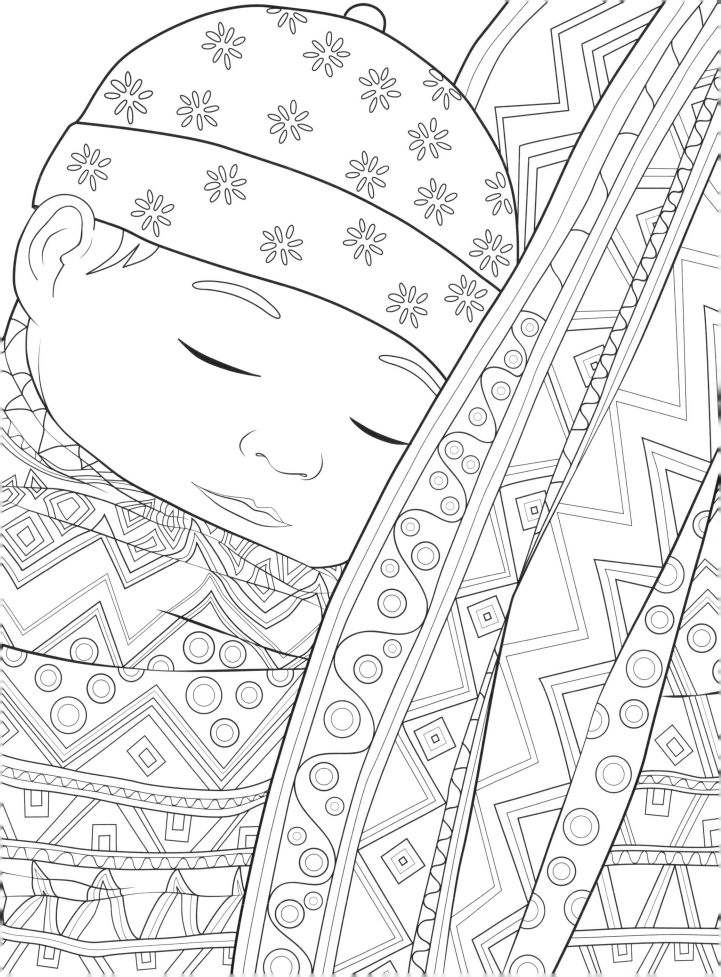

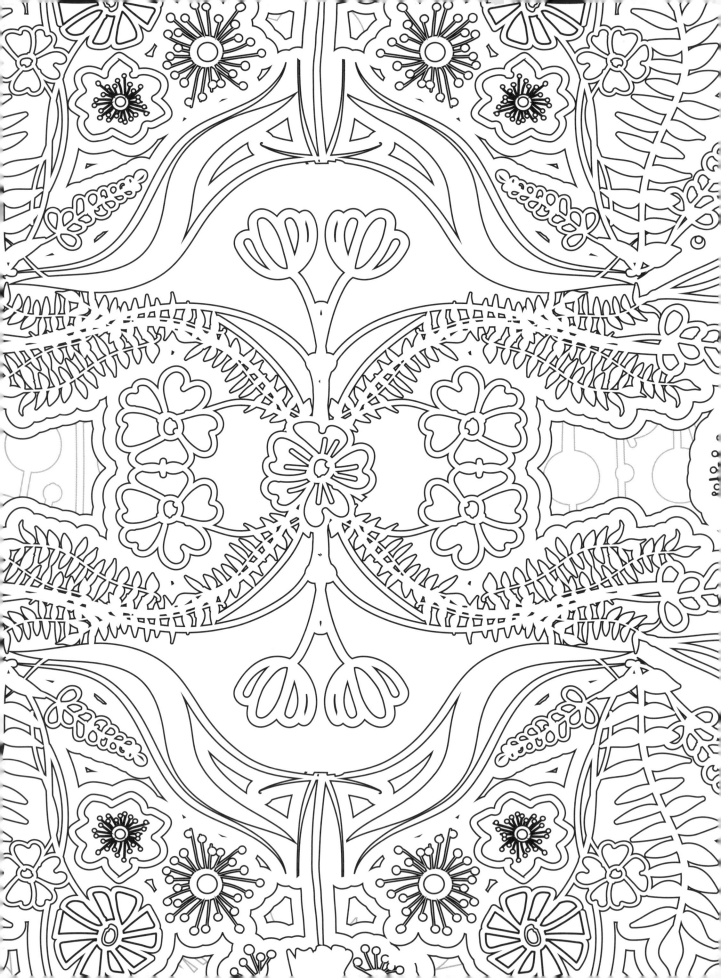

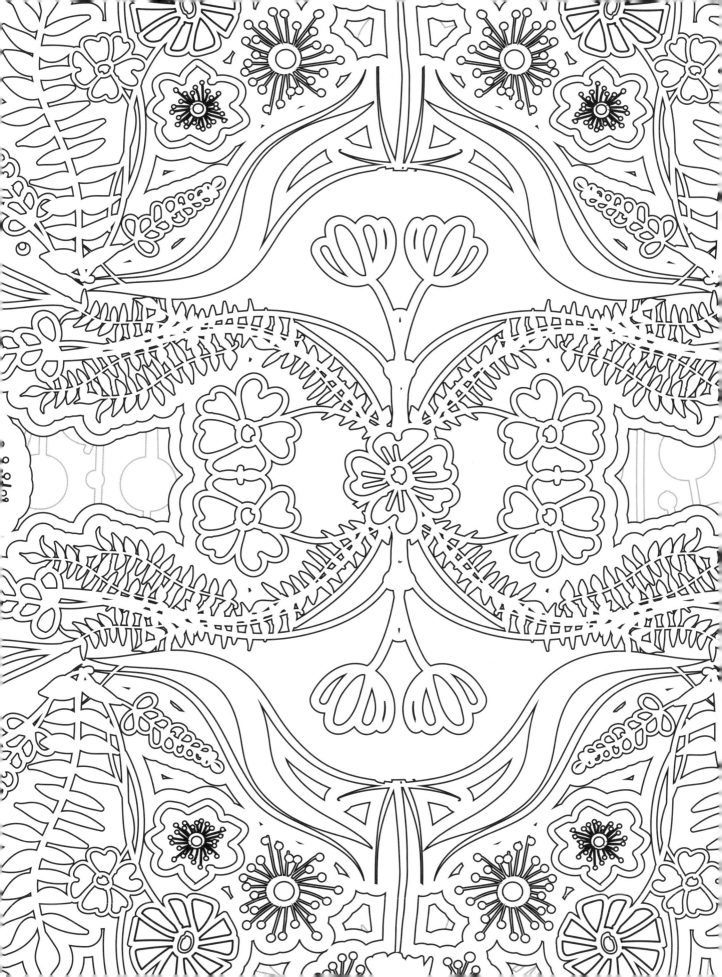

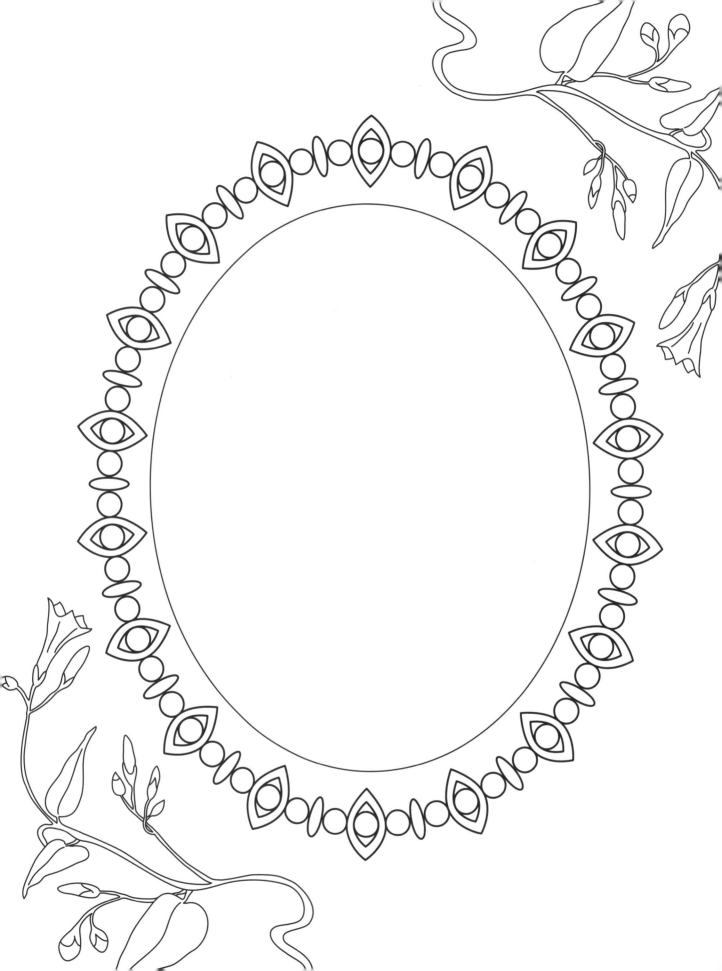

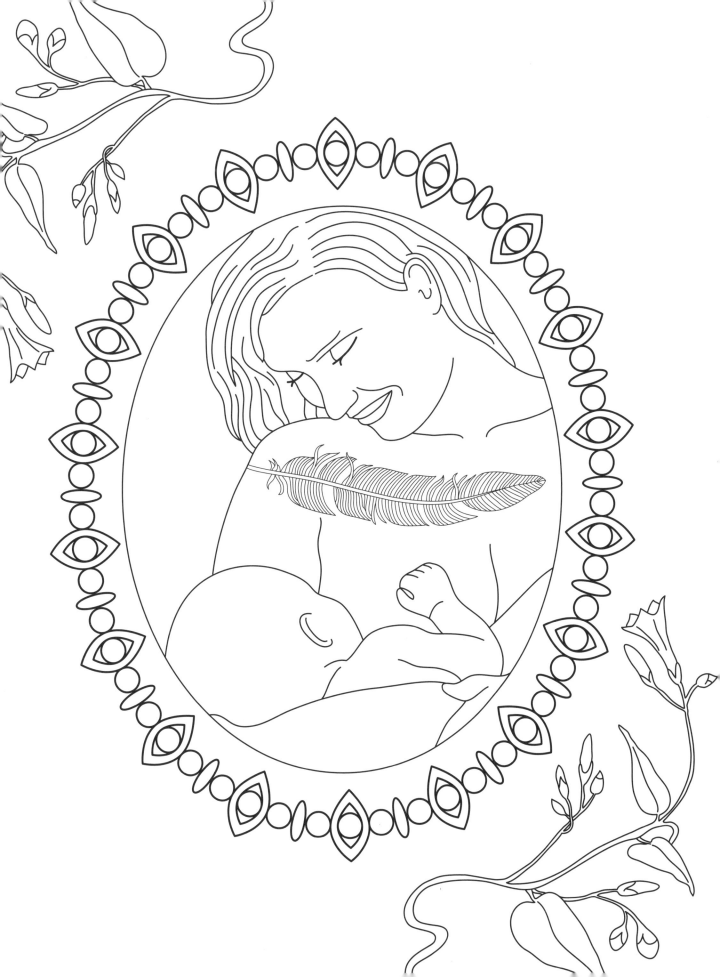

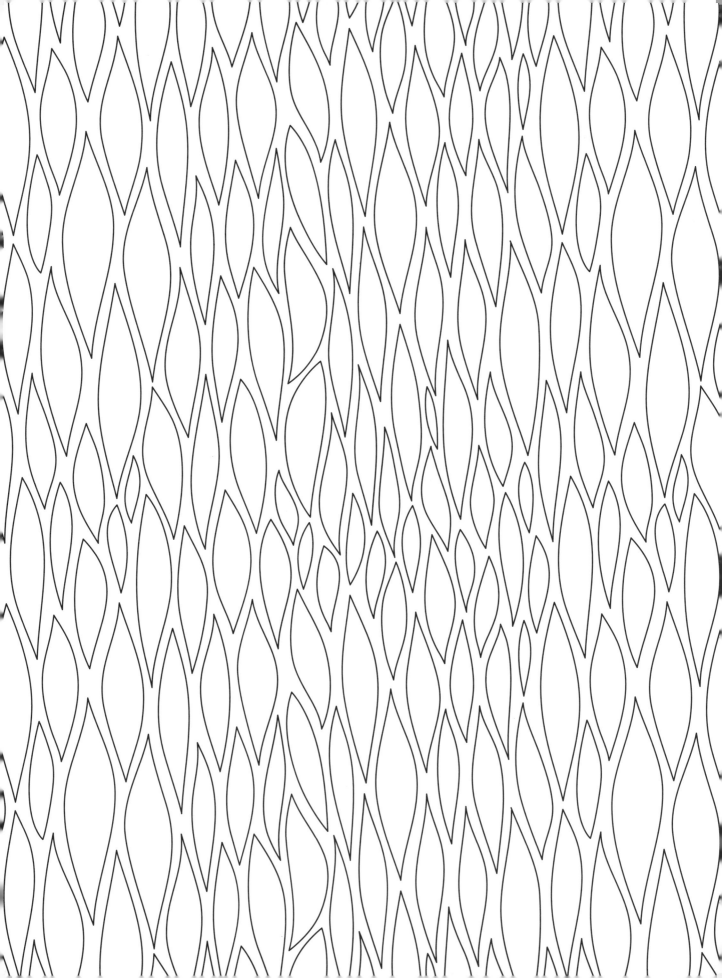

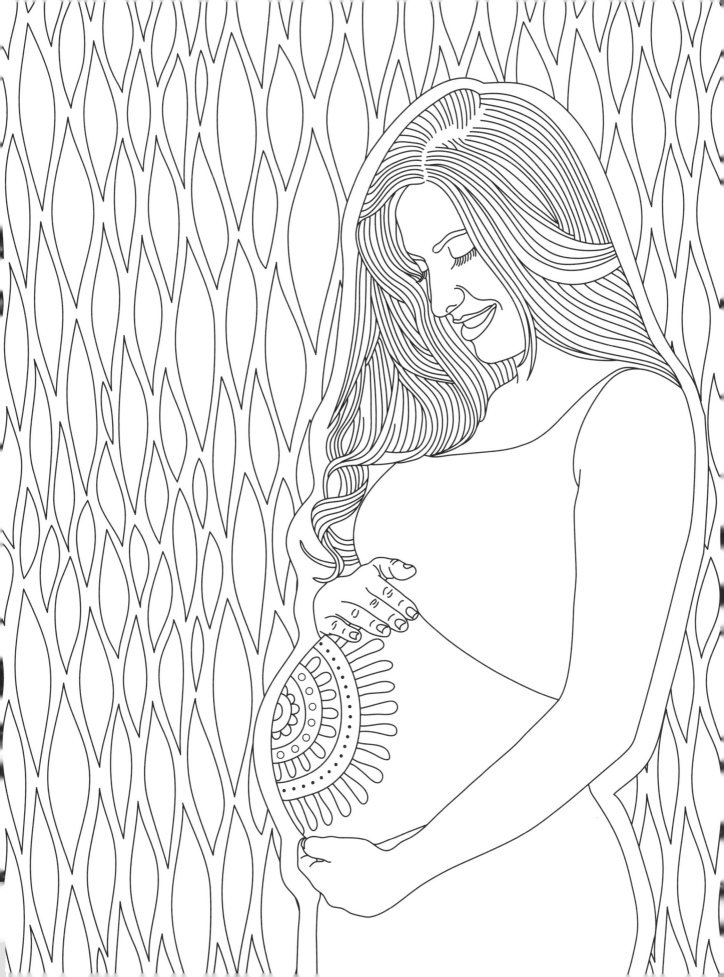

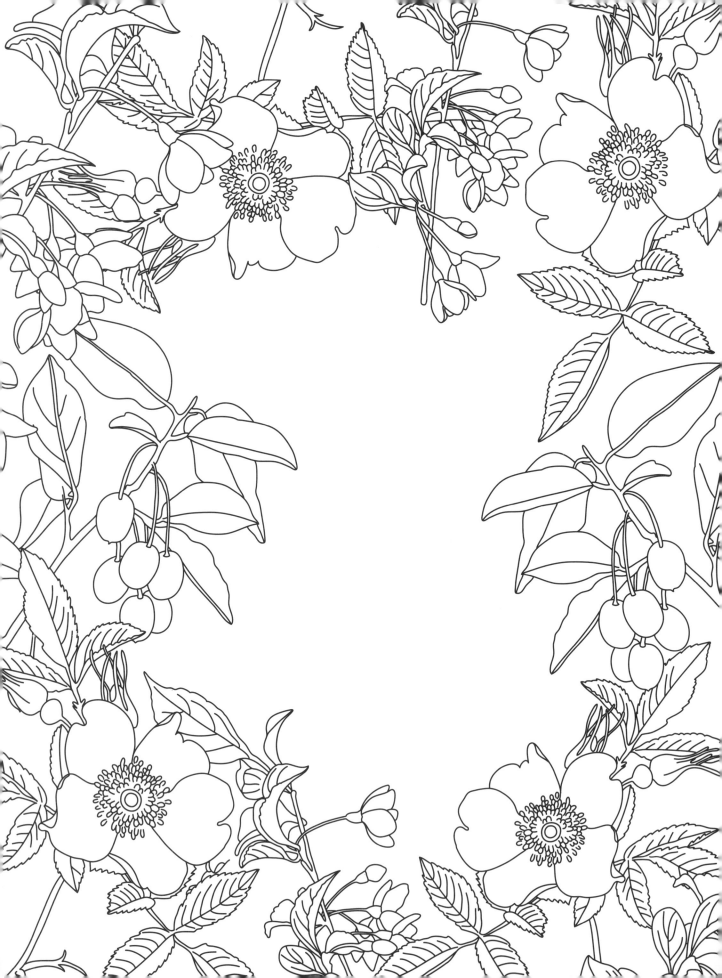

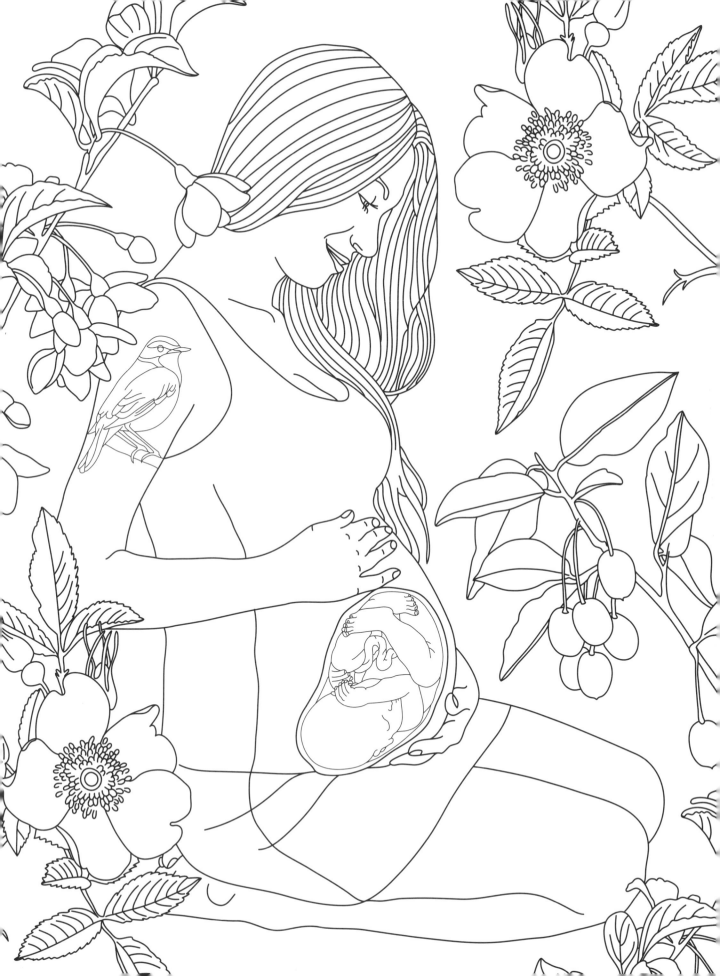

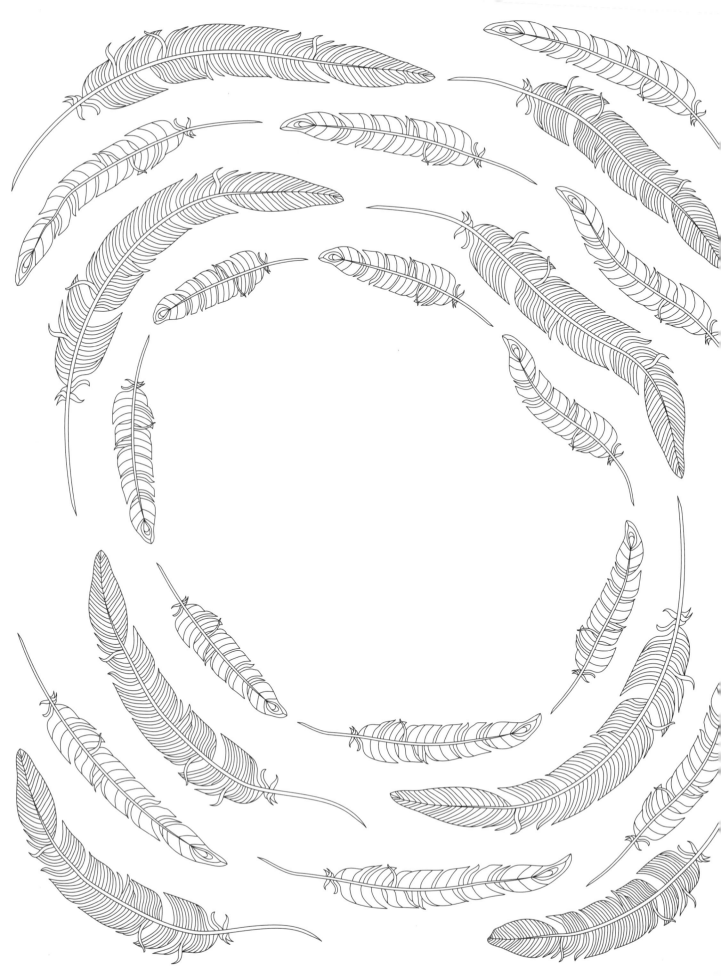

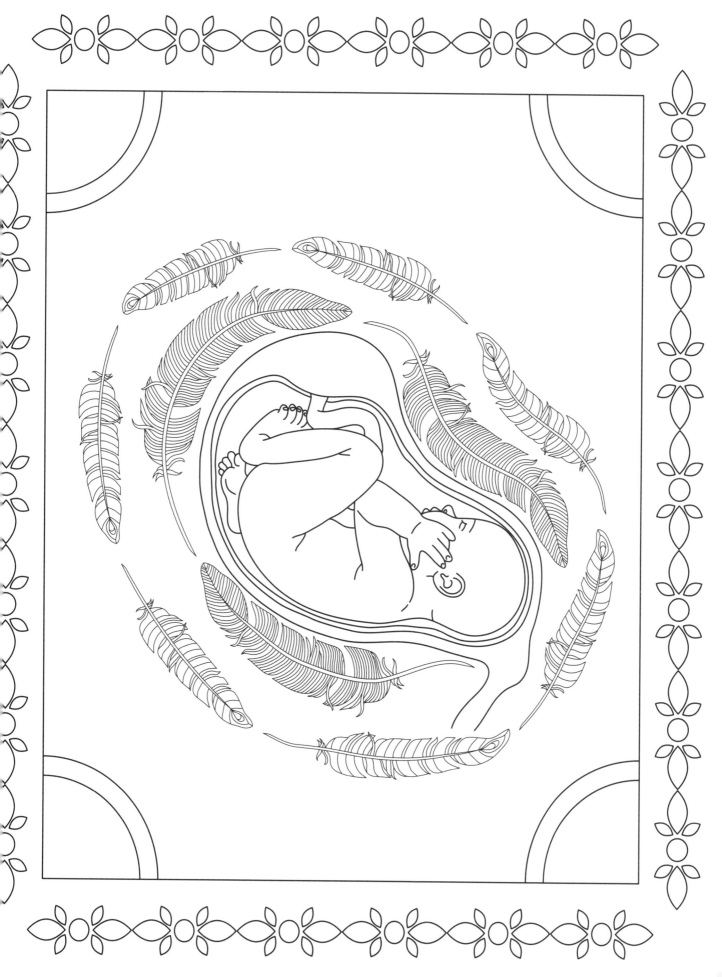

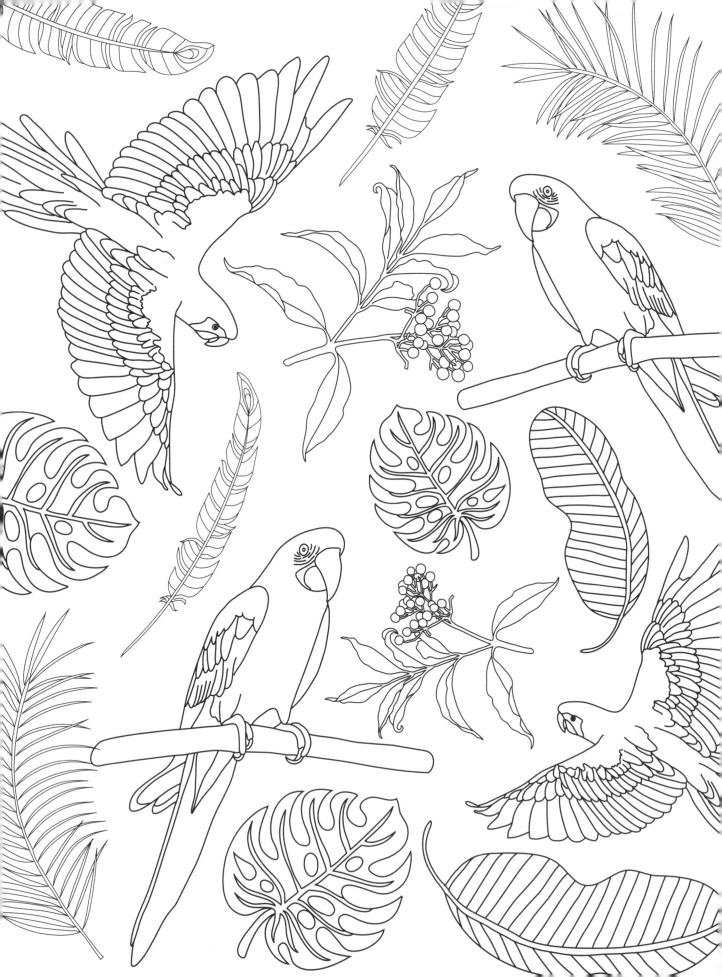

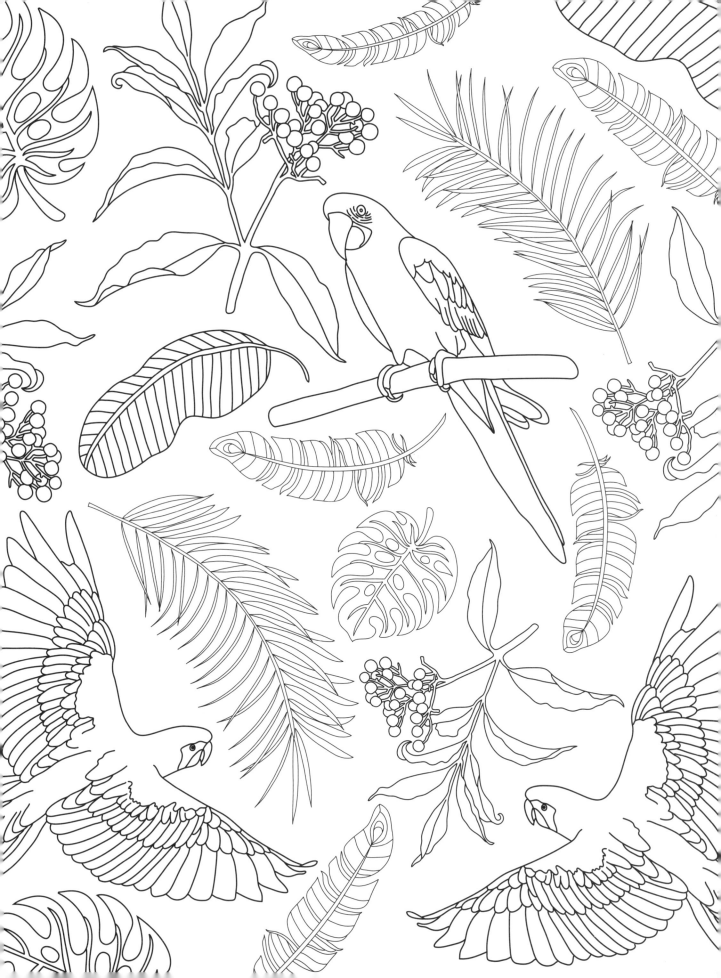

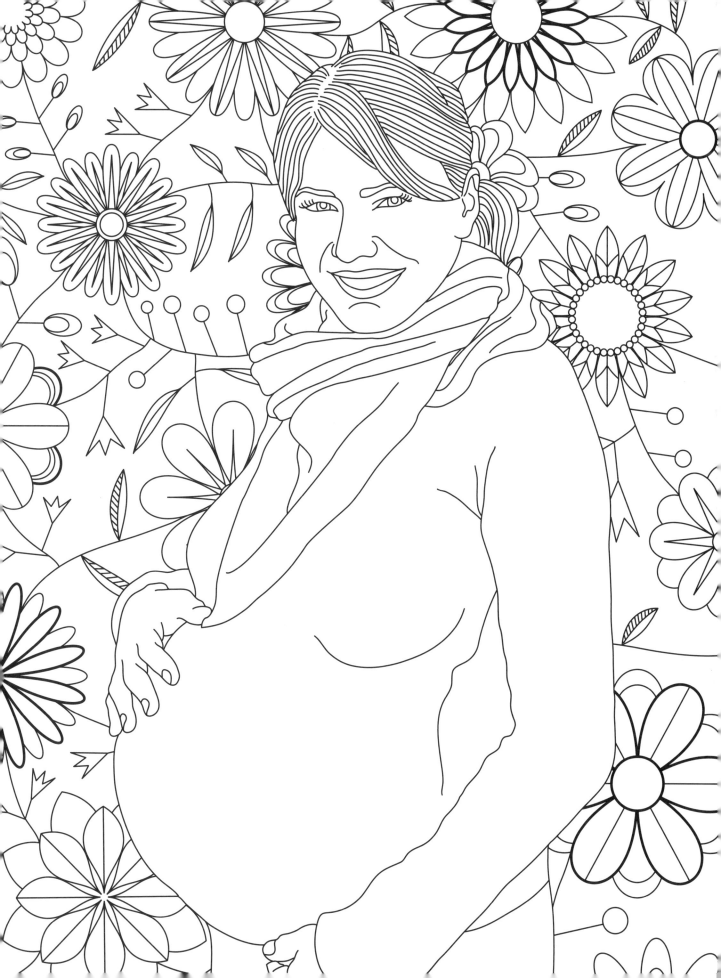

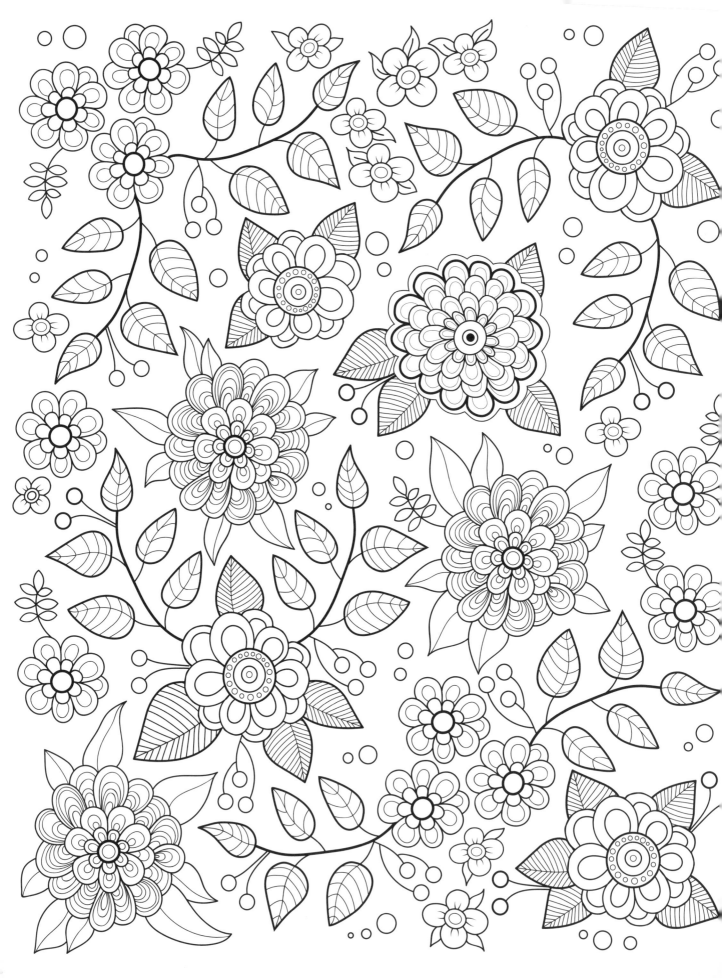

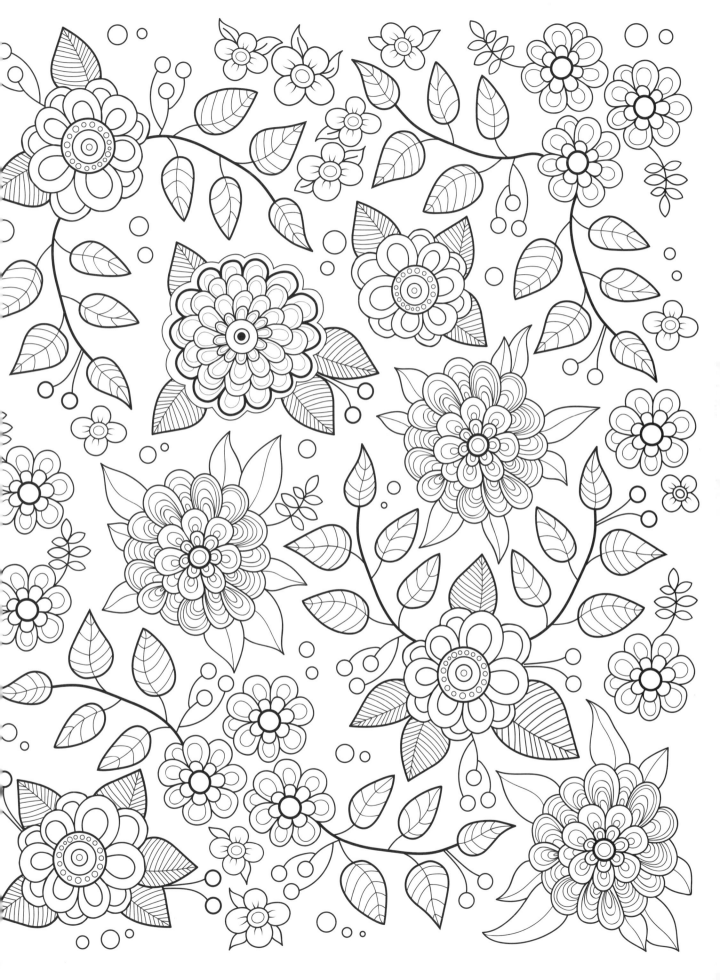

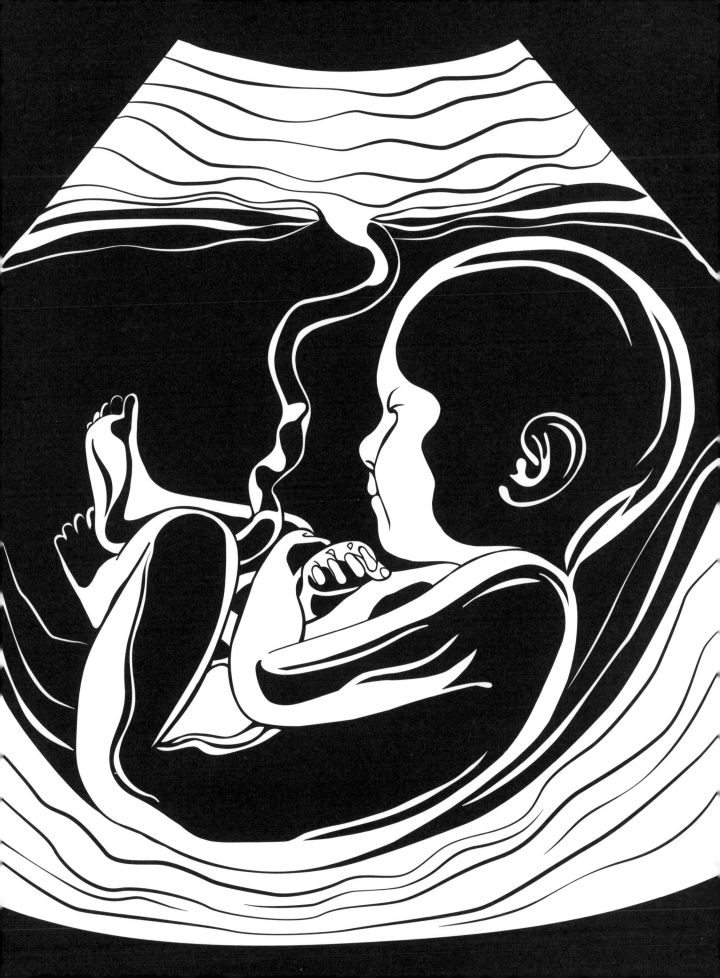

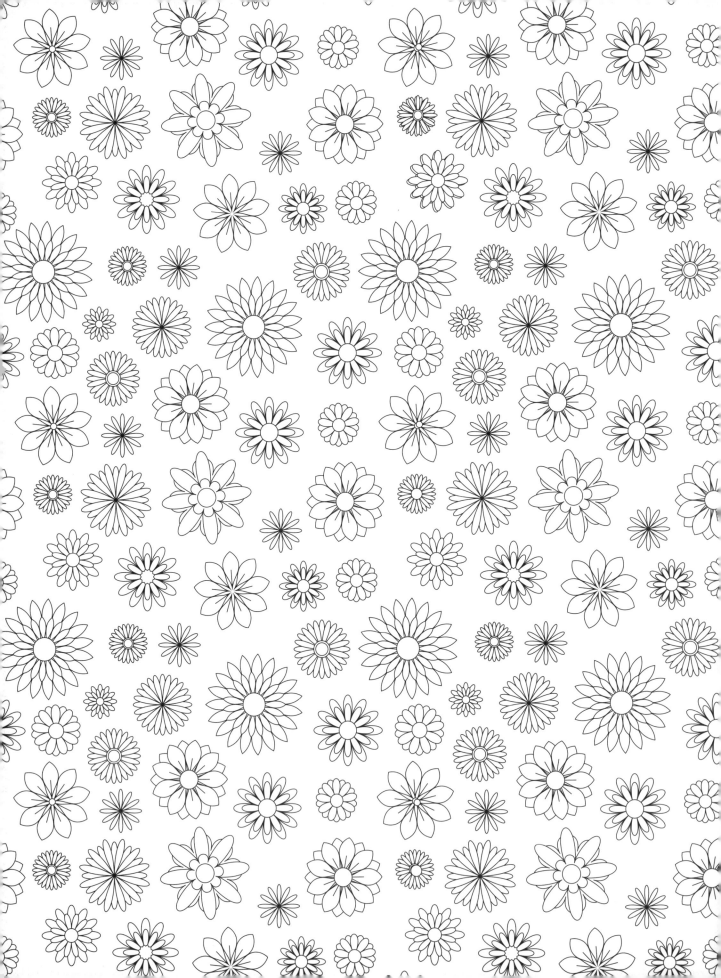

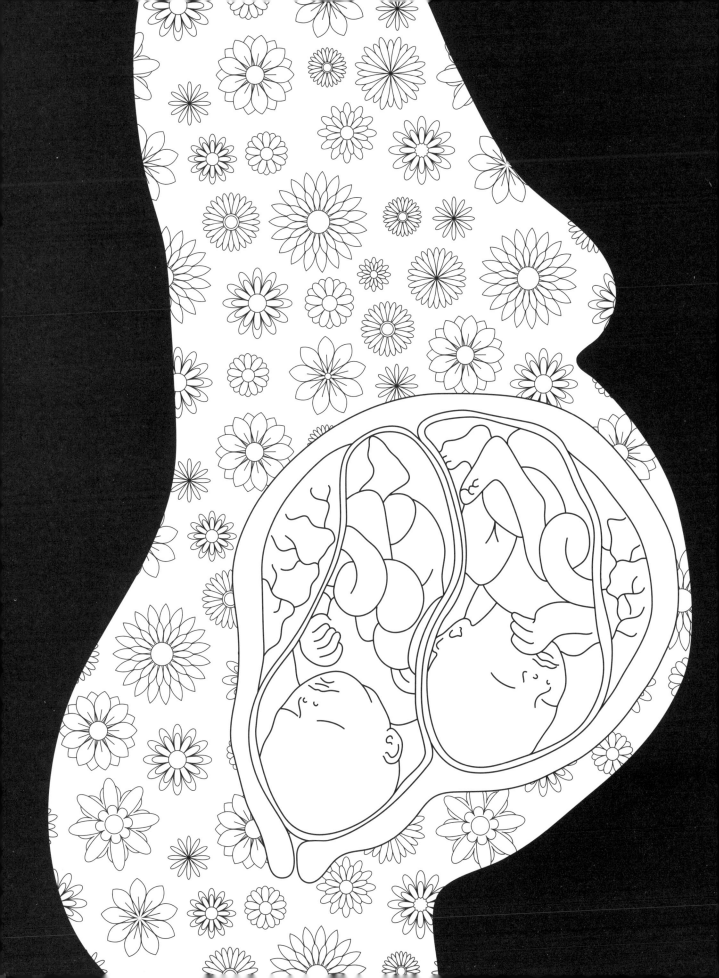

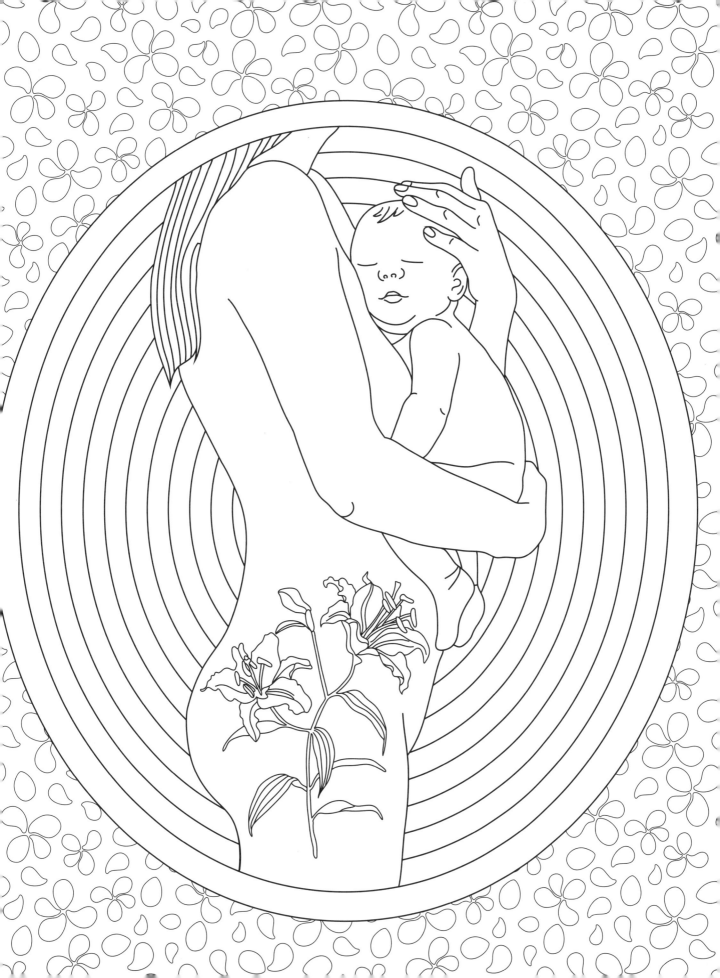

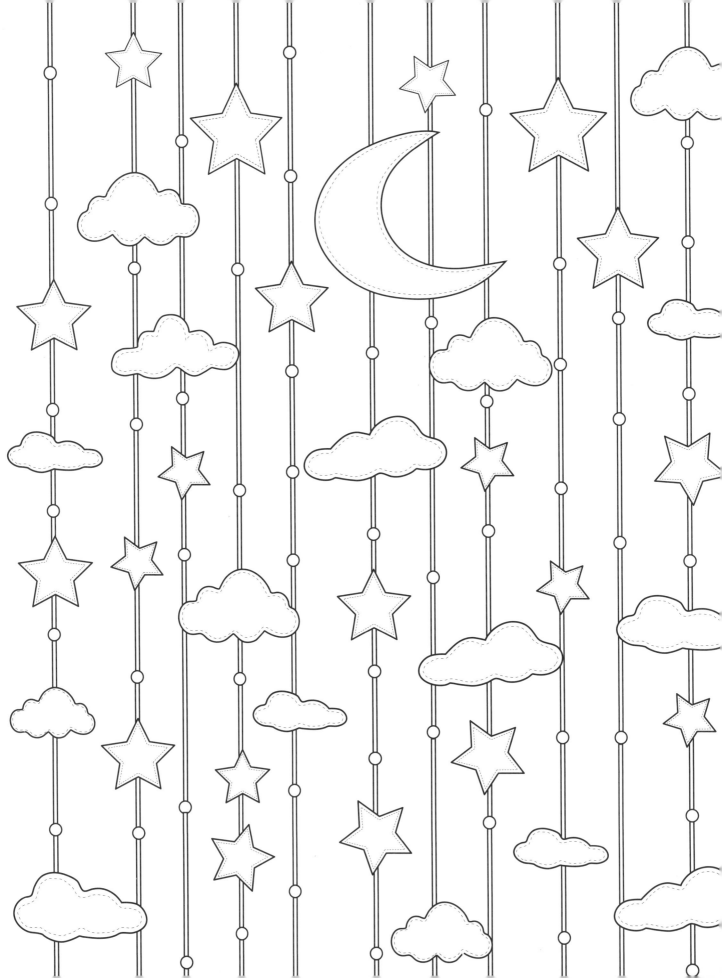

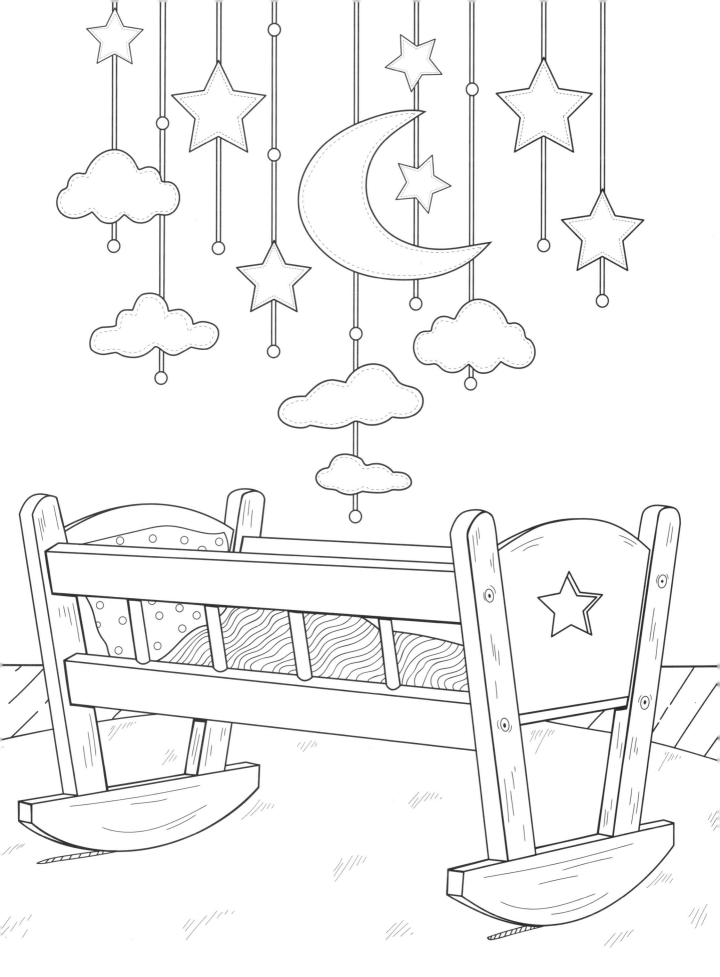

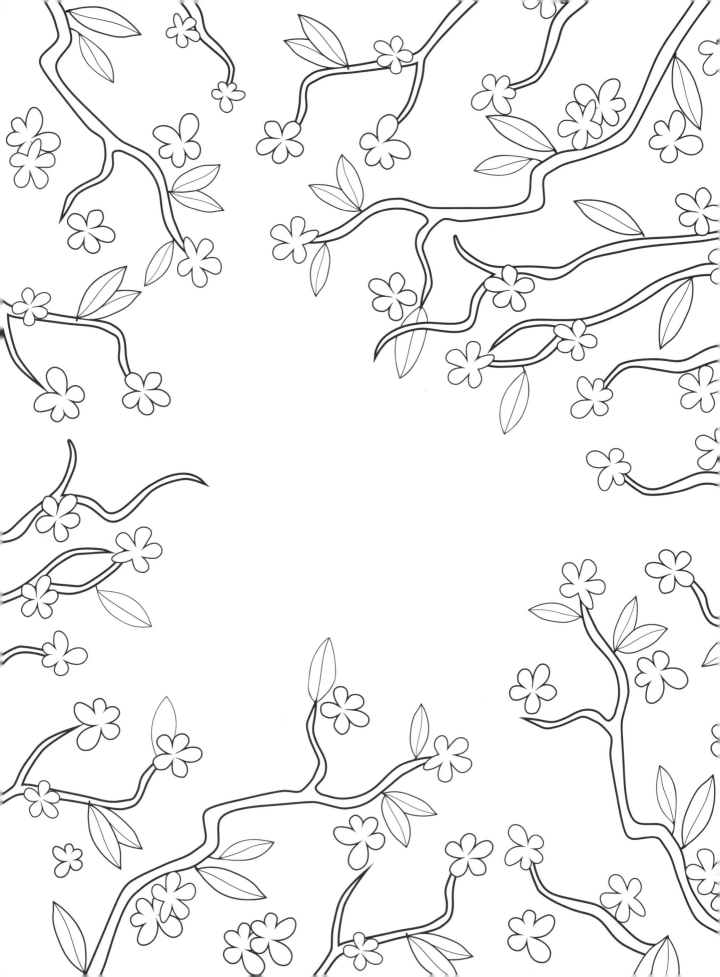

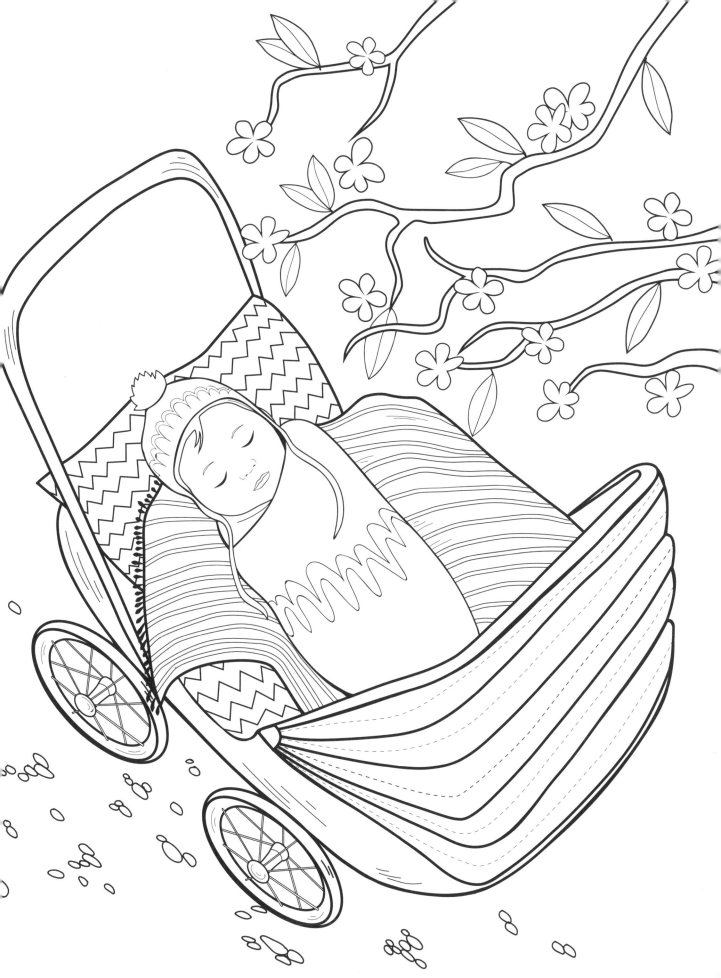

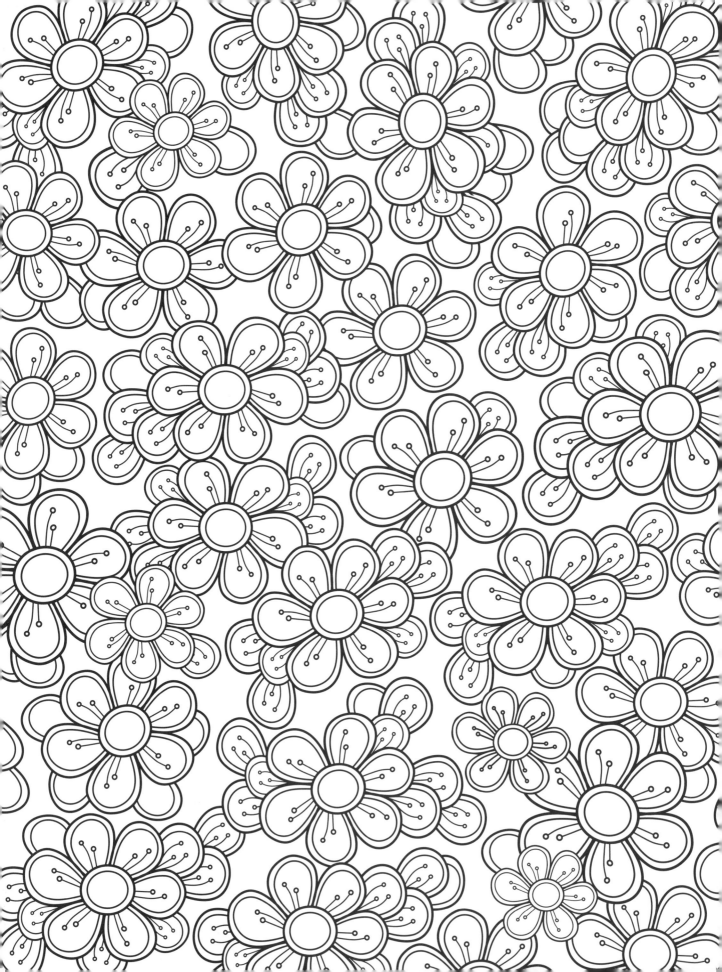

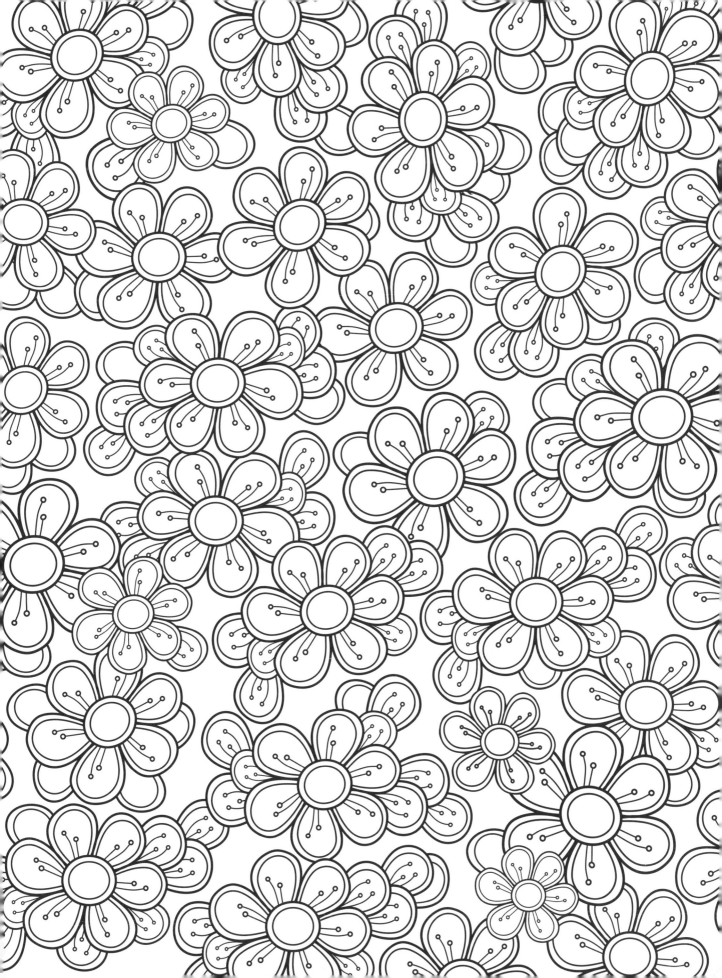

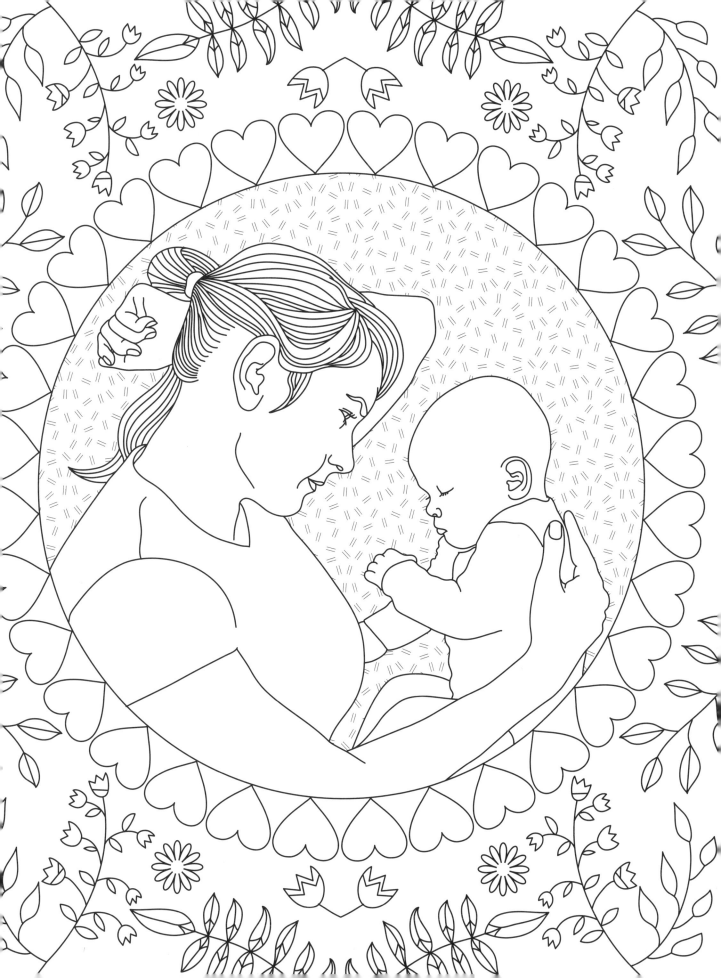

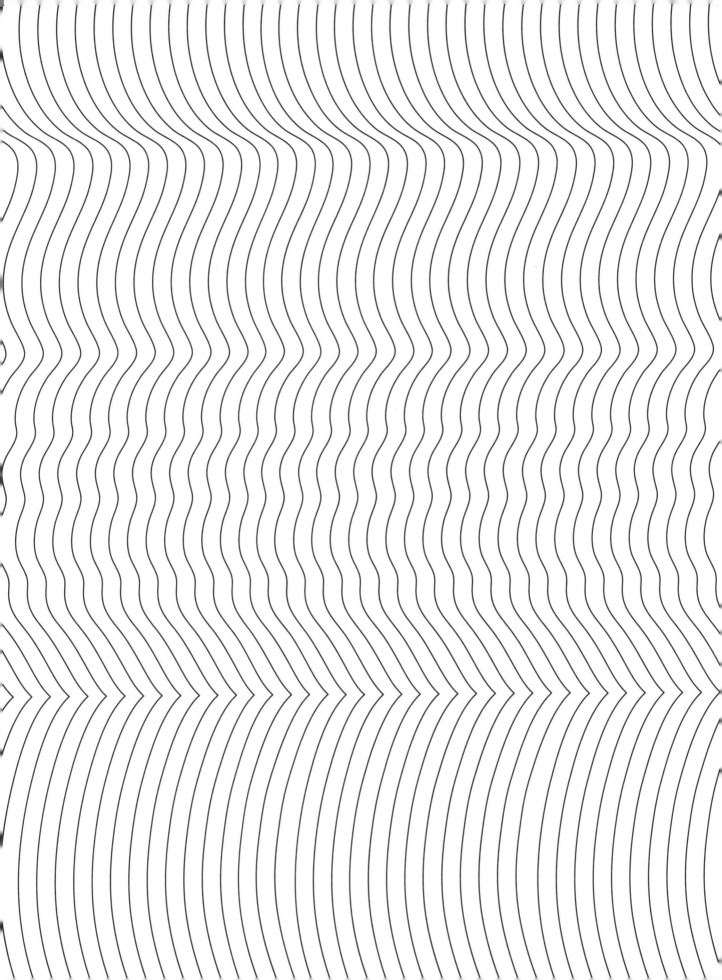

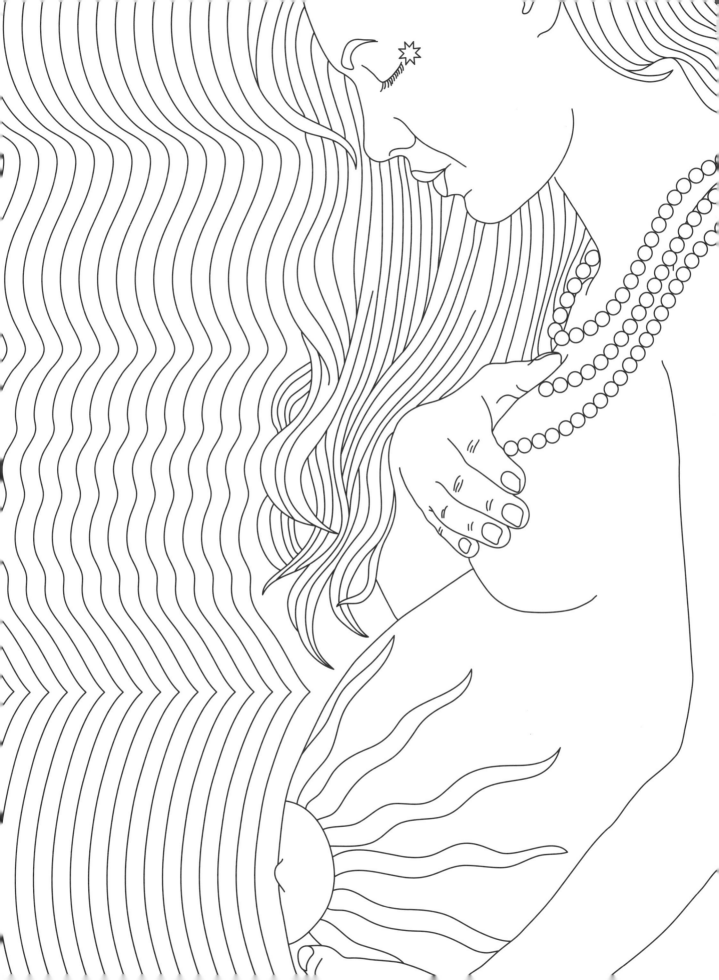

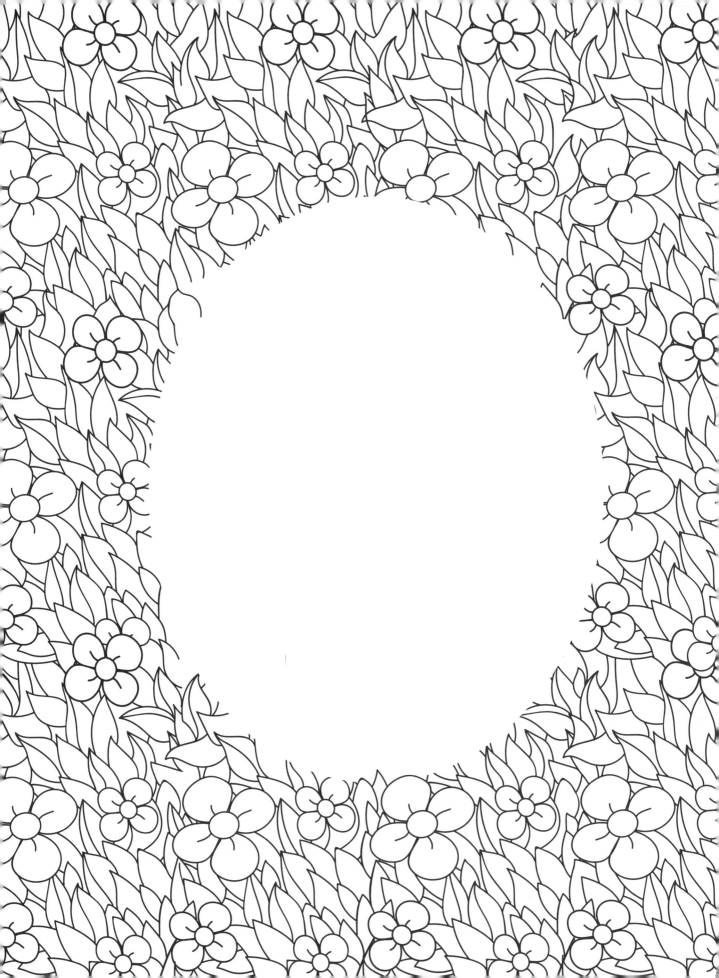

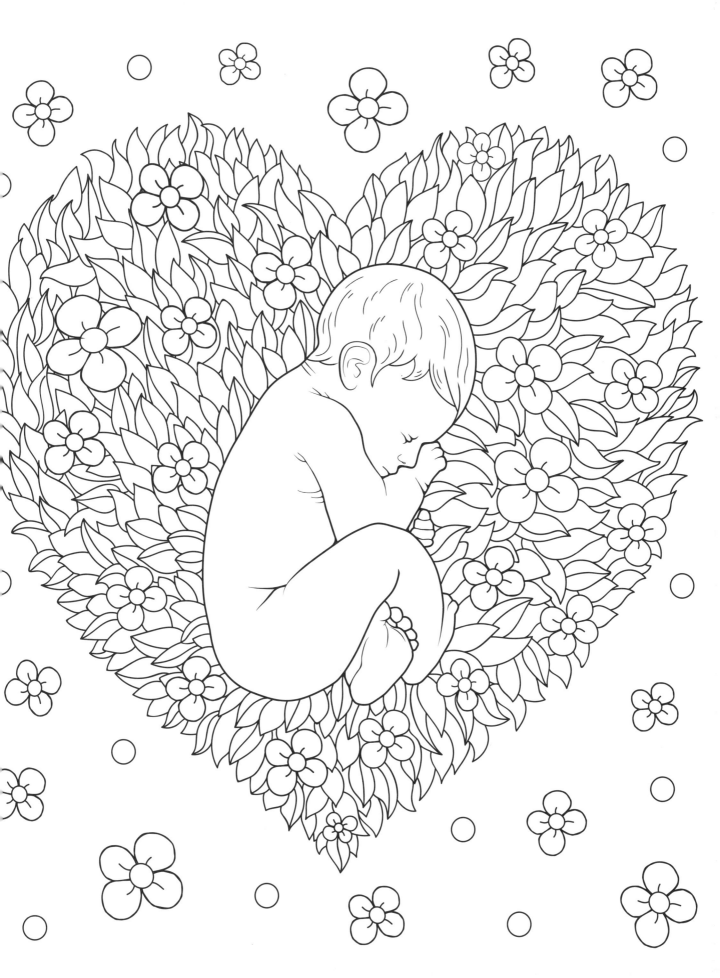

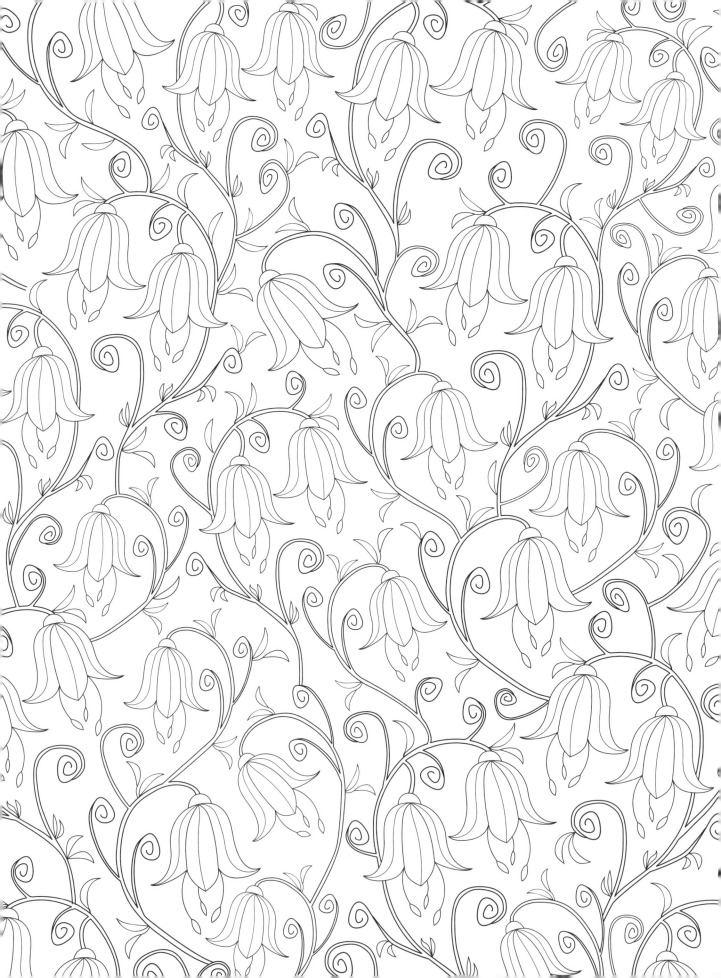

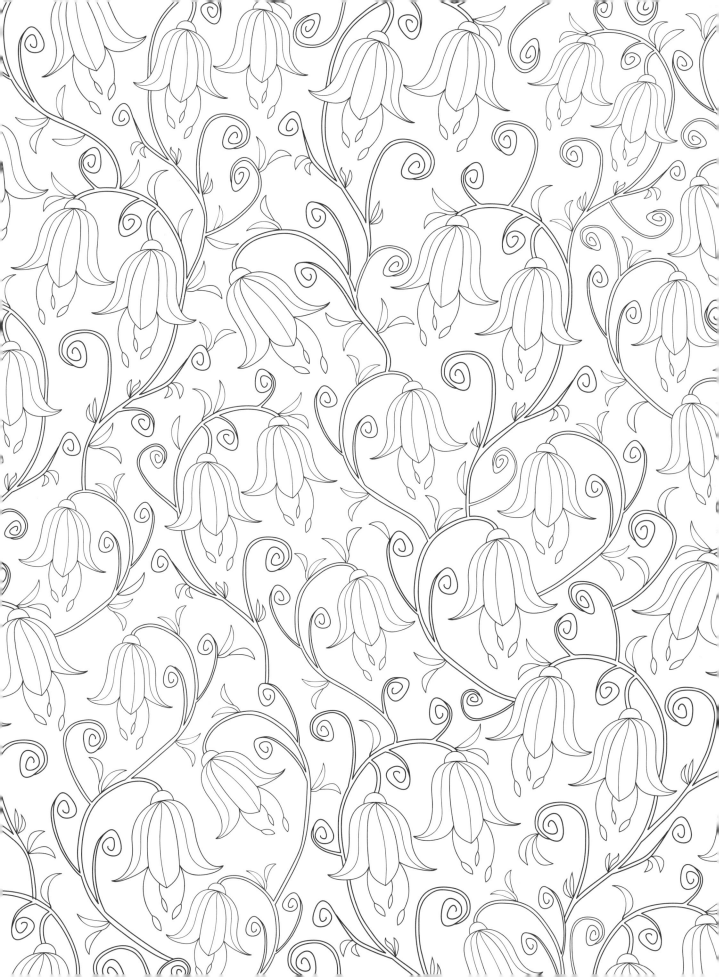

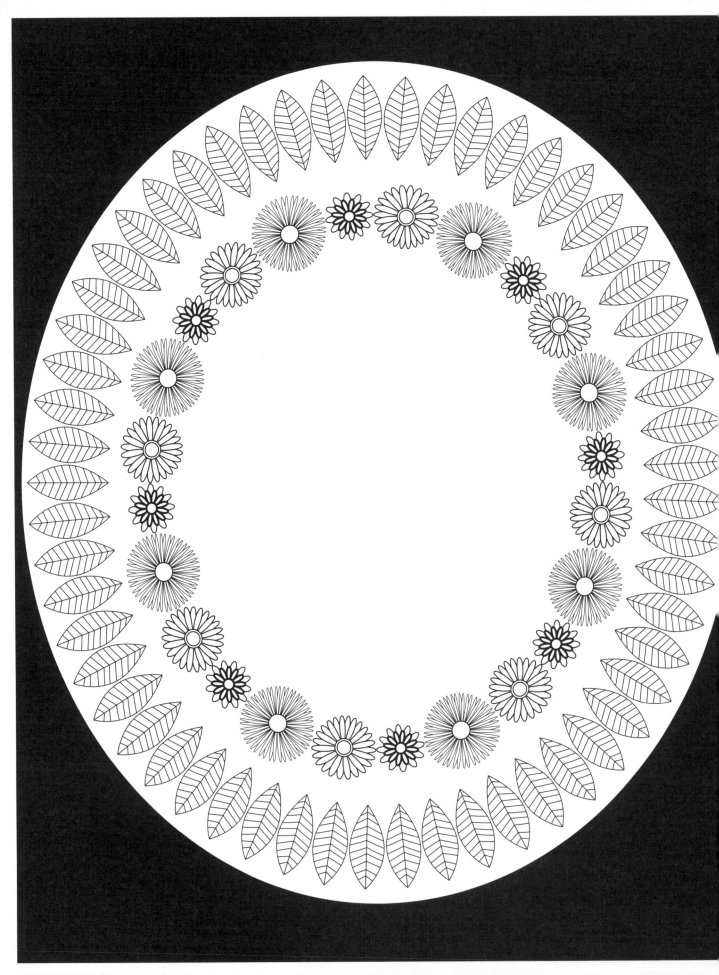

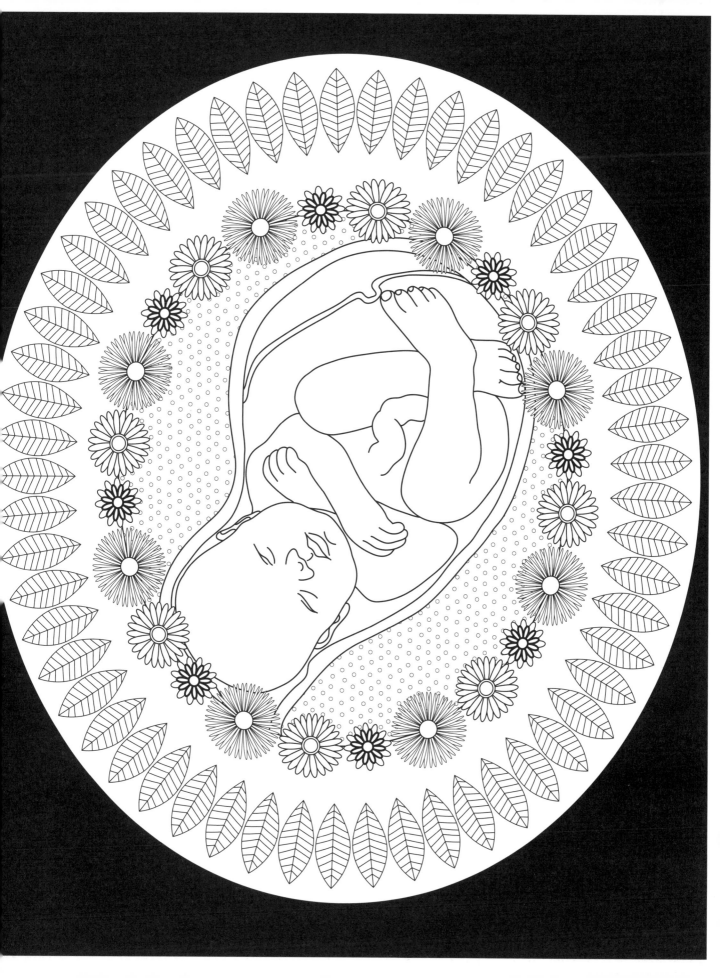

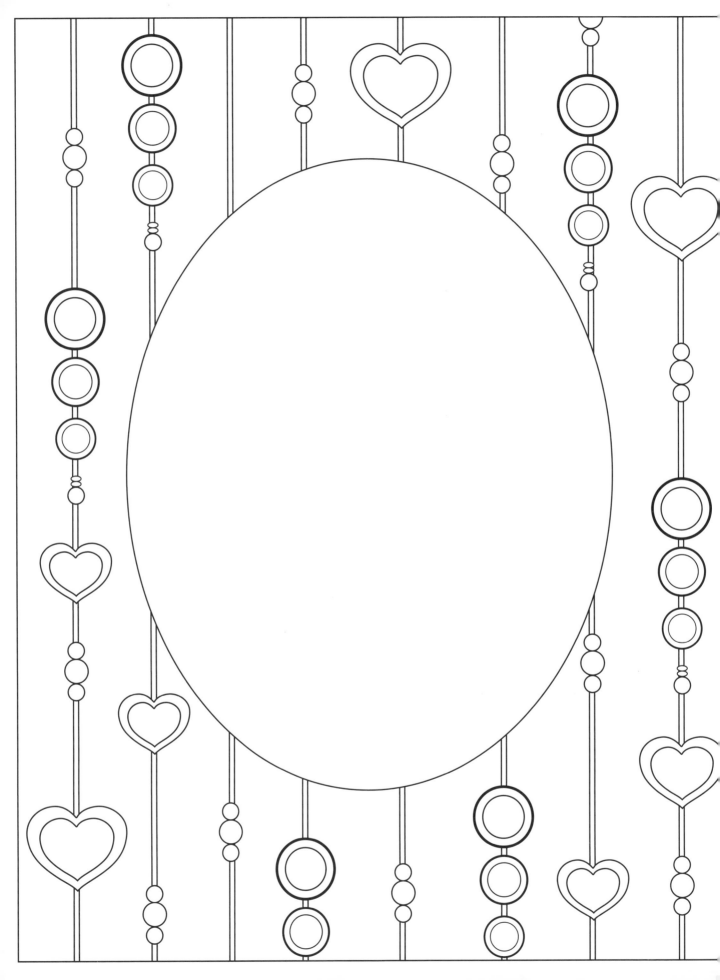

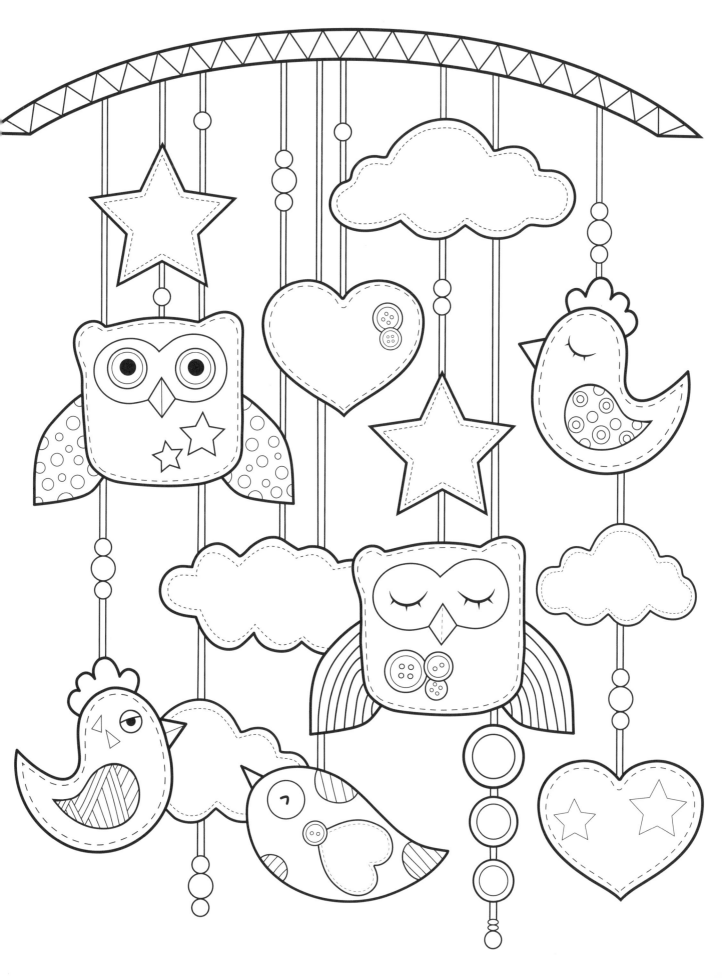

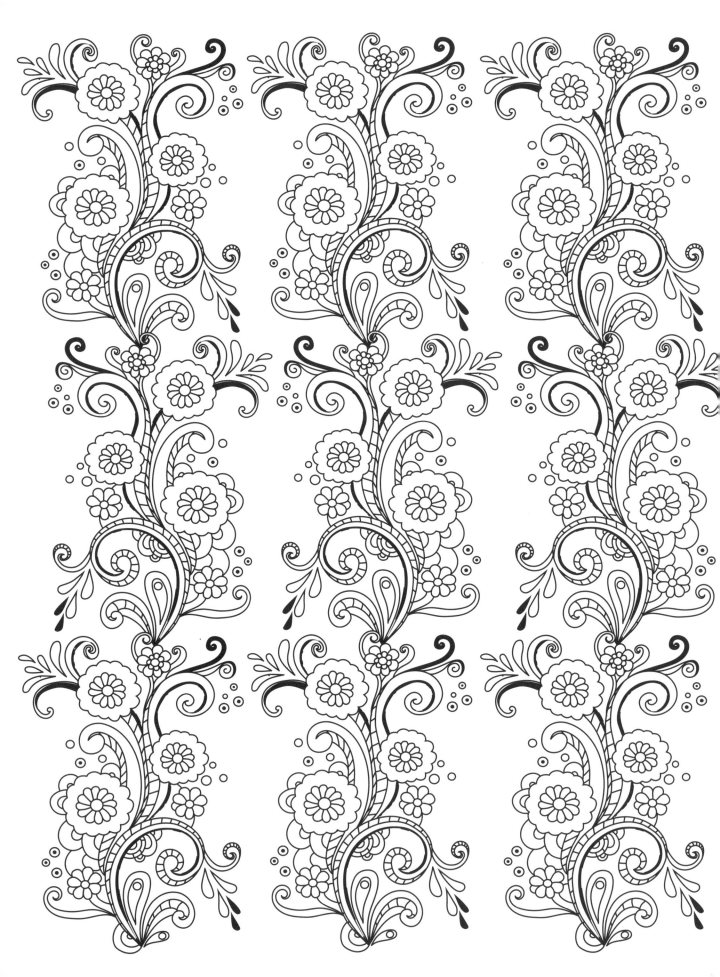

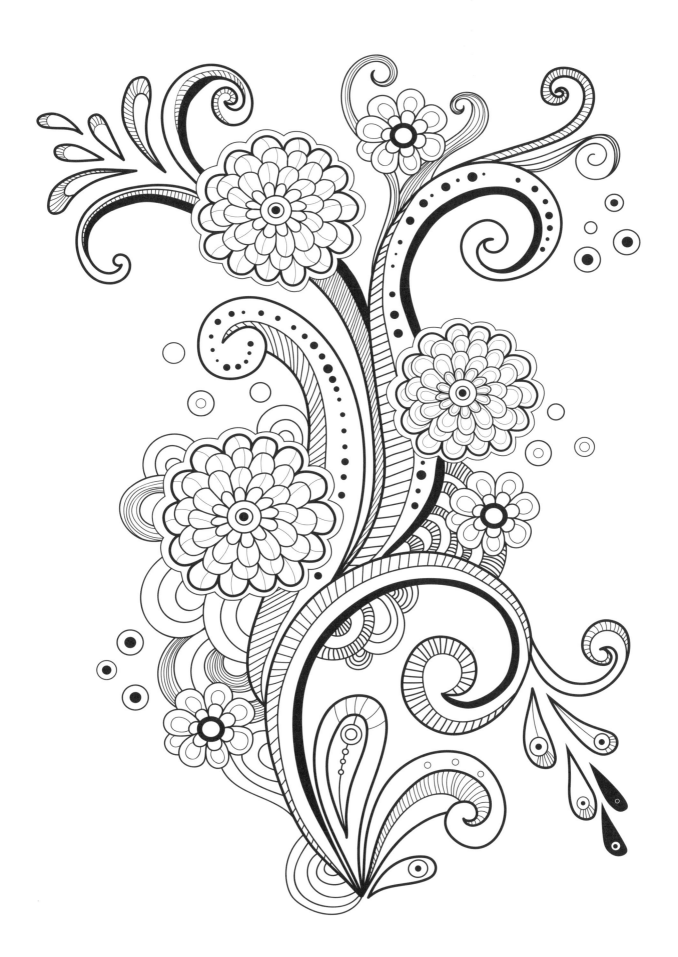

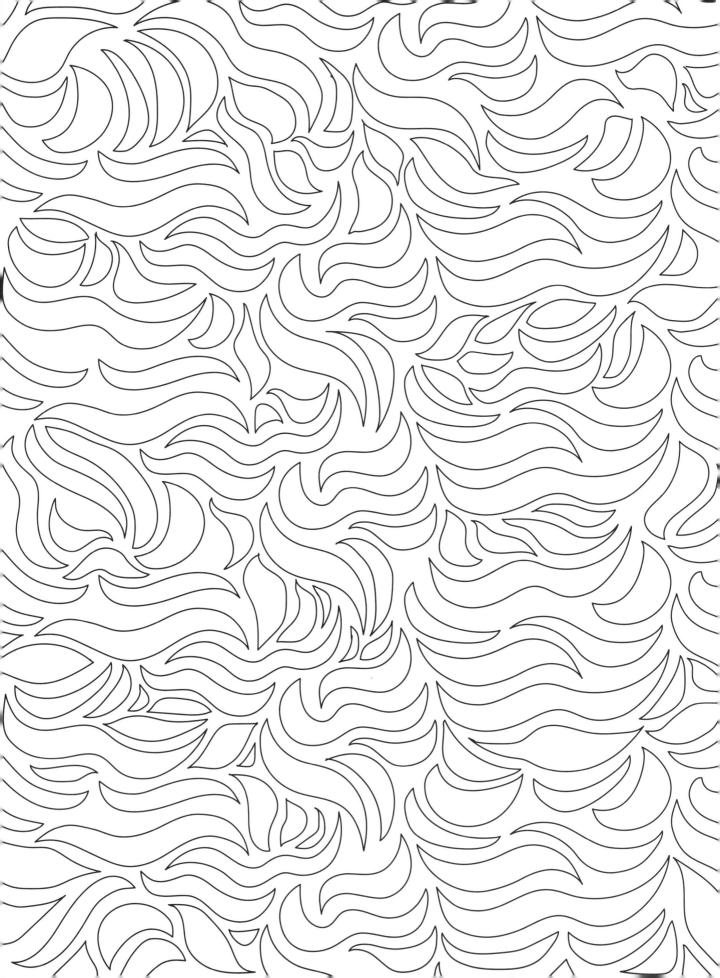

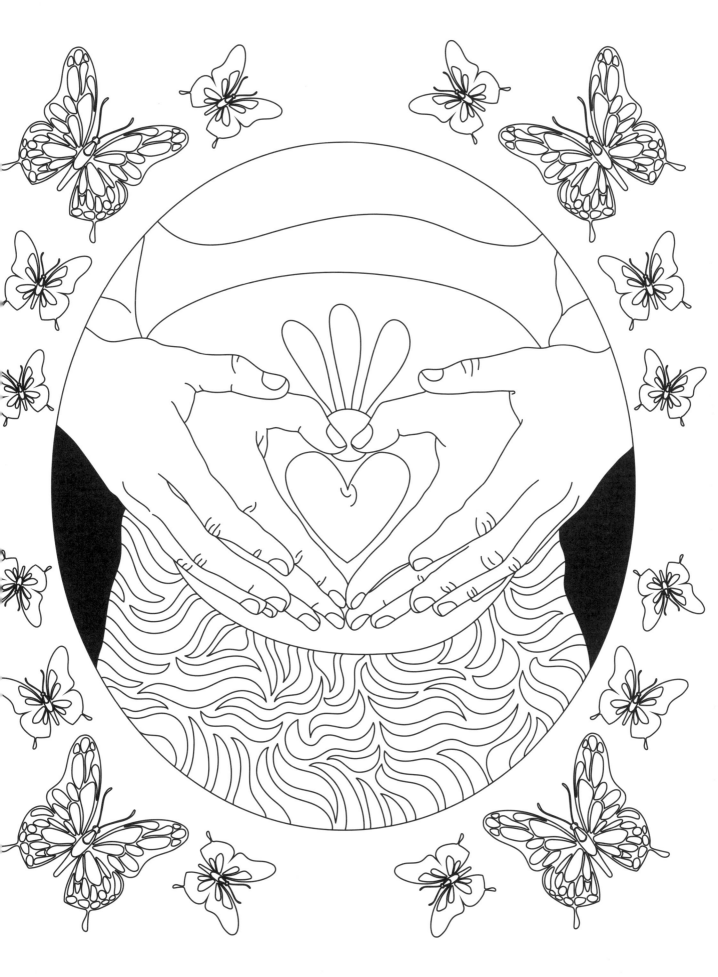

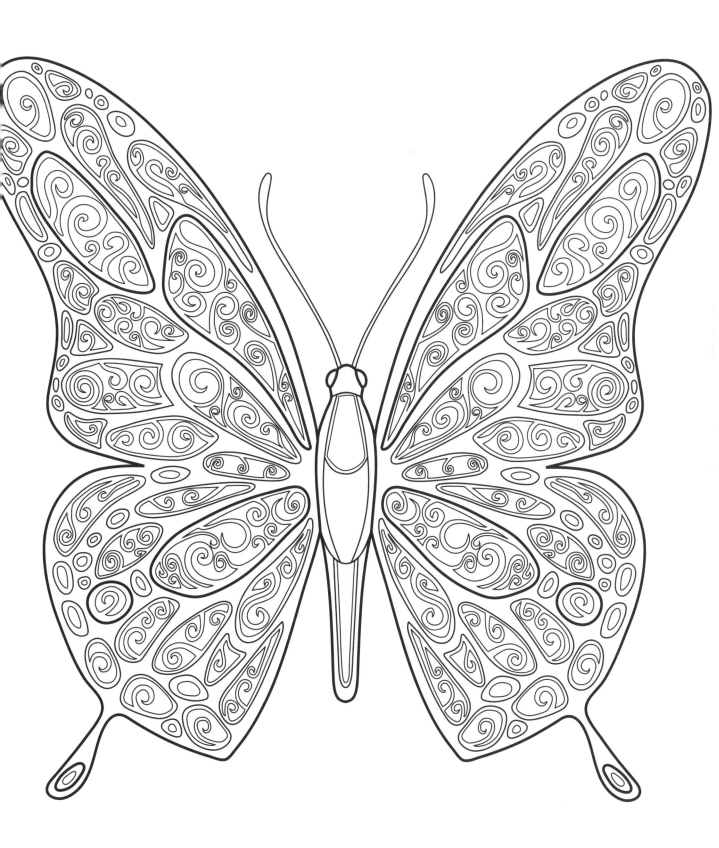

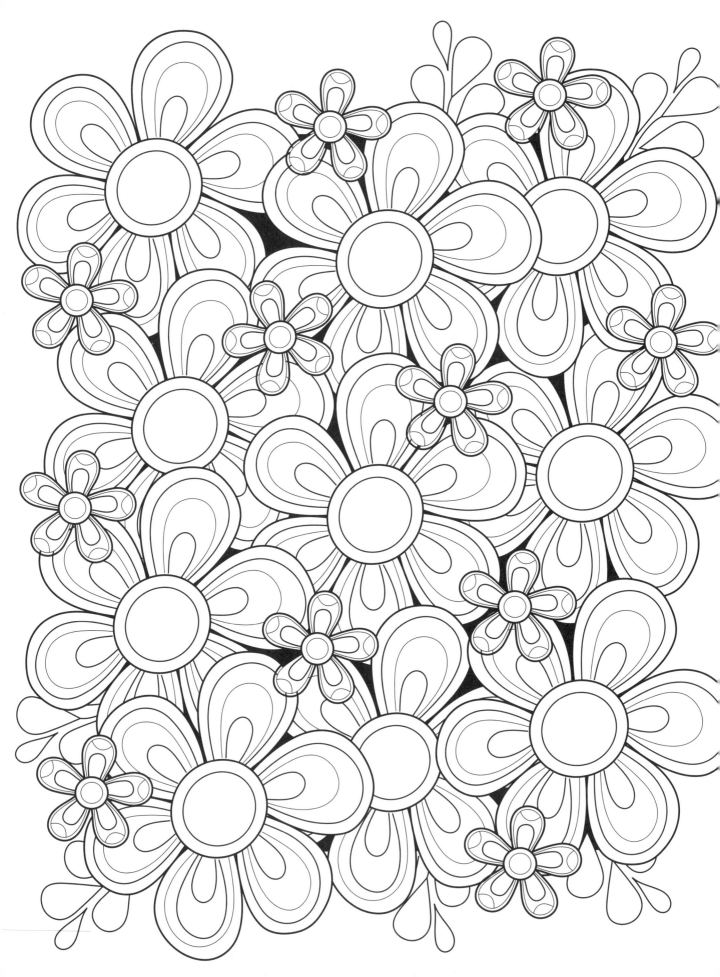

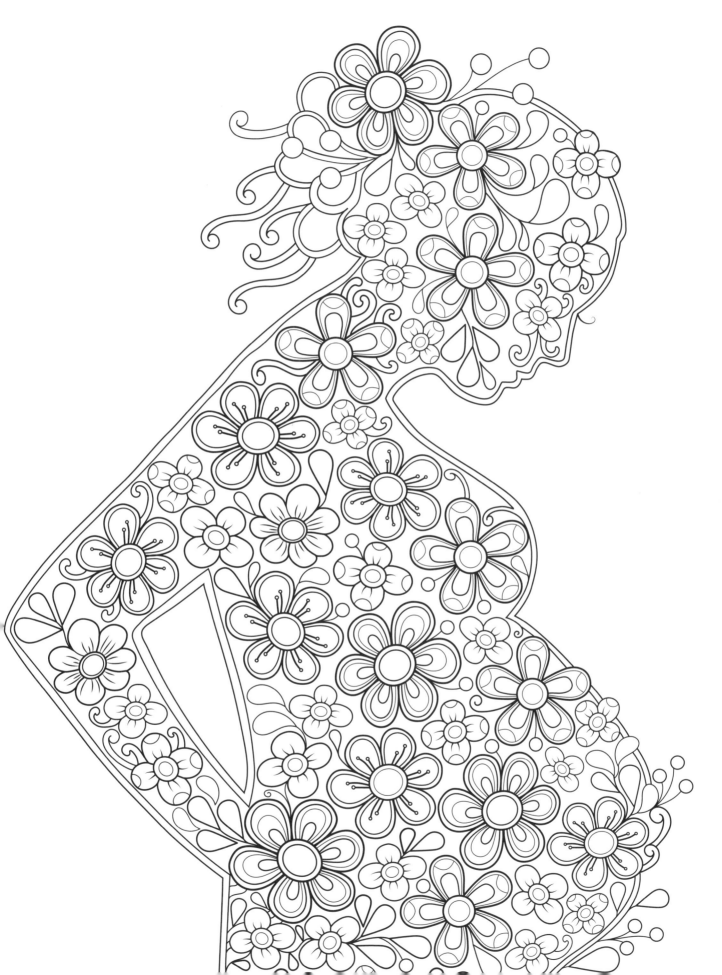

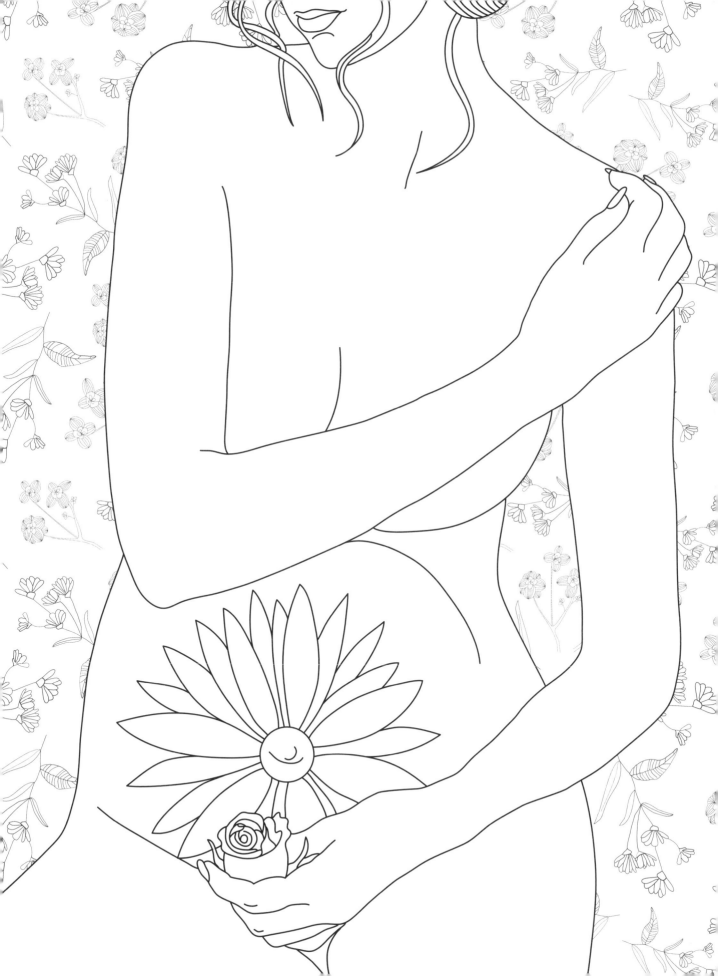

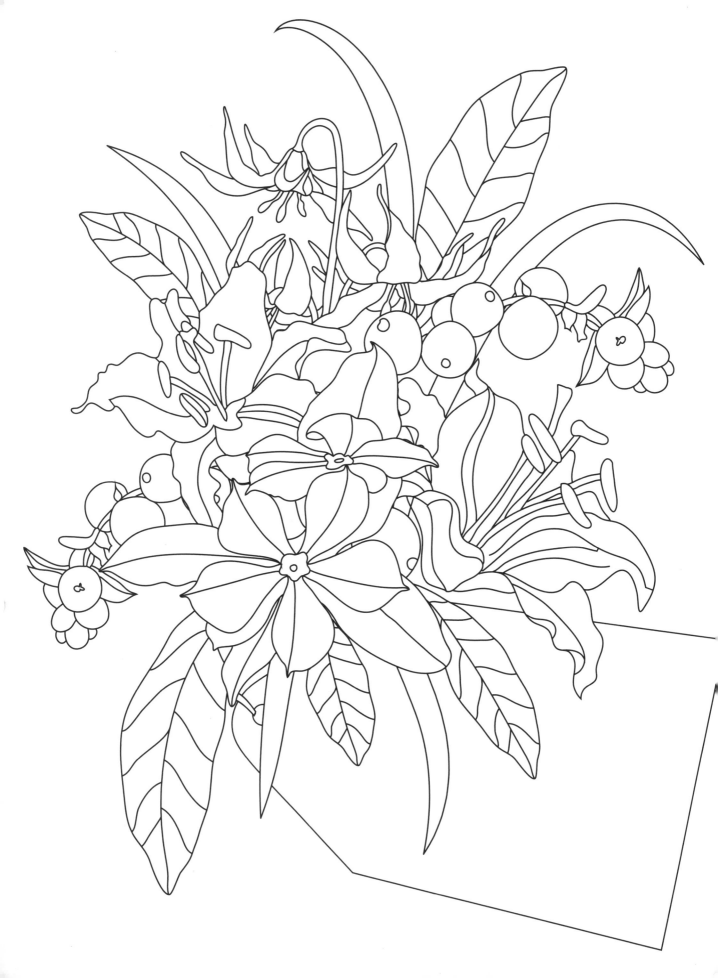